The Edible Fountain of Youth ™

"Eat the Way YOU Want to Look" ™

Author

Susan M. Poore

R.N., C.N.C., C.P.L.C., C.H.P.

Healthy Aging Expert

www.TheEdibleFountainOfYouth.com

First Edition 2016

The information herein is not intended to be a substitute for medical advice. This book and the content provided herein are simply for educational purposes, and do not take the place of medical advice from your personal practitioner. Every effort has been made to ensure that the content provided in this book is accurate and helpful for our readers at publishing time. However, this is not an exhaustive treatment of the subjects. No liability is assumed for losses or damages due to the information provided. You are responsible for your own choices, actions, and results. You should consult your personal practitioner for your specific medical and dietary needs.

Cover photo by Melissa Stokes @ Mack Visuals

Cover Design by Rob Williams

Edited by Gerri Shepherd

I dedicate this book to all of you...

To Dr. John R. Norman, a cardiologist for over 50 years and one of the most intelligent physicians I have ever worked with. Dr. Norman spoke of the unhealthy inflammation that occurs in one's body causing havoc, long before others rarely discussed it. I am incredibly blessed to call Jack, my dear friend for life.

To my parents, Jean and George Manske, who raised me to be strong and focused, with a foundation of love and understanding.

To my children, Chris, Jeni, Kiel and Ashley who are amazing adults now. They are blessing my life with beautiful grandchildren.

To my patients, colleagues, clients and close friends who inspired me to write this book, putting into words all my knowledge and love for living an incredibly healthy lifestyle.

To my husband Thane, who has been my biggest fan and cheerleader while on my journey helping to inspire others. You have always believed in me and what I was capable of, never doubting my abilities to do anything I put my mind to or any dream I had. I appreciate your support more than you know. Always have...Always will.

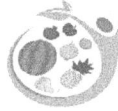

The Edible Fountain of Youth
EAT THE WAY YOU WANT TO LOOK

Contents

"Health is the greatest gift,

contentment the greatest wealth,

faithfulness the best relationship."

~ Buddha

Journey to Wellness...

"Surround yourself with people who are better, smarter, happier, stronger, fitter, wealthier, friendlier, funnier, and wiser than you. Hang around people who are more successful, more disciplined, more family-oriented, more connected, more experienced, more energized, more loving, more relaxed, and more generous. Learn from everyone."

I read this on the internet and loved it. Not sure who to give the credit to but they are some of the best words of wisdom I have ever read.

As we are on our journeys to live well, improve and maintain our health and live the best life possible, we need to surround ourselves with others who bring out the best in us. It's all a part of healthy aging.

My passion is to share my knowledge, while learning from others along this blessed journey we call life. I say "life is good" all the time whether I am having challenges or successes. Our minds are powerful and will believe whatever we think or say. Every day of my life, I wake up and if I can set my feet down on this blessed earth for one more day, I repeat to myself "life is good!"

I dedicated this book to several people. For those who really inspired me to write it with passion and to share with the world my knowledge and excitement about nutrition and living well as we age.

Over the years, I have met patients who needed to change because their health was affecting them in so many ways including financially and within their relationships. Together, we worked hard on returning them to a healthy state, and then maintaining it. Eating healthy is and always will be a huge part of your fountain of youth.

I am so honored to join in with all the medical practitioners that have stood their ground for decades, stressing the importance of nutrition and how it can heal and improve one's health and quality of life. When all their colleagues were prescribing numerous drugs and doubting the effects of a plant based diet; they were inspiring their patients to change what they put into their engines (gut) which in turn cured many of them of their illnesses. They have proven that a person's diet can and will dramatically effect even hereditary diseases. I am blessed and in awe of them and will be forever grateful for all I have learned.

 A few times throughout this book, I will repeat myself in different ways, this is purposeful because not every one reads a whole book, they may pick a few chapters that interest them or skim through it. There is a message in each and every chapter and I hope to inspire my readers to take to heart what I have to share.

Ask yourself, as you read through each and every chapter - what information can I really grasp and throw into my "Edible Fountain of Youth Basket?' When you are done with this book, then return to your "basket" and get started from there.

If you are reading this book for the first time, my wish for you is that you will bring many of these positive habits into your life, so that you too, are aging gracefully and with the best health possible!!!

Eat the Way YOU Want to Look...

Namaste'

Susan

"The way you think,

the way you behave,

the way you eat,

can influence your life

by 30 to 50 years."

~ Deepak Chopra, MD

Chapter 1

What does "Anti-Aging" mean?

Anti-aging is not just about the lotions and potions that may promise you age reversal. Aging has been studied continuously for hundreds of years. Today, we find out how to take care of ourselves through others habits (good and bad) and the results that are recorded.

Aging is a multibillion dollar industry. There are more lotions, potions, juices and concoctions out there than ever before. Unfortunately, none of them can give us "forever" or many would be consuming it!!!

I do not refer to myself as an "anti-aging practitioner". I am certainly not "anti" (meaning against) aging as it is part of our circle of life we cannot change. But we can extend our lives and do it well with health and happiness IF we are willing to follow the right path.

Consciously working on your health and then maintaining it is not the easiest thing to do in a world where there are fast food restaurants around just about every corner. But we do know that with the right information, the right guidance and certainly a lot of effort on our part, we can age gracefully.

If not an anti-aging expert, then what is my "title"? Quite frankly, because of my education, training and experiences I have, I consider myself a "Healthy Aging Expert." You see, I know that we will ALL have a birthday every single year that we are on this planet. I also know that most of us celebrate our annual milestones either feeling blessed or lucky as we age. Would we like to live forever? Maybe yes, maybe no. We just want the time we are here to be looking and feeling our best.

My passion in life is to really - Impact, Influence and Inspire. Leading a healthy lifestyle results from living well day after day. We now know that we can live into our 70's, 80's, 90's and possibly into our 100's. More and more people reach age 70 than any time in history. The "baby boomer" generation is huge.

Let me ask you, do you want to be the 70-year-old that has been in a nursing facility for the past 5-10 years OR do you want to be that 70-year-old who is teaching the exercise class at the health club? *What we do today, we pay for tomorrow, good or bad.*

I tell my patients that if someone announces a "study," don't assume the results will work for you specifically. What most people don't know is, when results of a study are announced you need to research it before moving forward with the recommendations. Studies can have as little as 3 people in it or 3,000,000 in it. It could be done in a different country. There are so many variances. When people hear about a study that allows them to do _____ (whatever), and that's something they like – well of course they want to believe it's good for them. I clearly follow the studies and research that are very reputable and have strong evidence. Rest assure, what you read in this book is proven healthy aging tips and suggestions.

As you read through the rest of this book, I want you to picture yourself at 70, 80 or 90 plus. What do you look like? Where do you live? How active will you be? Don't just "hope you make it", put the odds in your favor!

Could you work really hard on your health and still have issues later in life? Of course. But perhaps something hits you at 70 that would have occurred possibly 10 or 20 years prior. We are human and humans have challenges. I opt to create the healthiest body possible to help fight against those challenges.

My goal is to teach you how to prolong your optimum health with early prevention and of course early detection. Even if you are reading this book today at age 50 and have not taken care of yourself very well, realize that our bodies are very forgiving and with a great plan you may be able to gain back what you have lost. You never know until you try.

Healthy aging rocks!

Let's do this with grace and enjoy every moment…

"A healthy attitude is contagious

But don't wait to catch it from others.

Be a carrier."

~ Tom Stoppard

Chapter 2

Why I wrote this
"Healthy Aging" book...

I asked myself several months ago. "Why write a healthy aging and lifestyle book when there are thousands of books like this out there?" I will be honest with you; I was highly encouraged to write this book by hundreds of people over the past several years.

This book is written for ANYONE (vegans and non-vegans) looking to improve their nutrition; for those who strive to be well; and for those planning ahead. If you want to feel and look good regardless of what your calendar year reads - then this book is for you!

Thru my private practice and with the hundreds of seminars I have done, I have met people who did not add a plant based diet into their lives because quite frankly they did not know where to start or they did not understand the tremendous effects that plants could have on their health. My goal with this book is to inspire you to learn that every effort you put in will all be worth it. Your entire body and mind will thank you...

Just about everyone knows what to do with meat, and how to cook it. People get stuck on what to do with veggies unless it's a potato or corn. So I hope to inspire Vegans and Non-Vegans alike into a healthy lifestyle. Even for those who chose to eat meat, this book is full of so much information that will enhance your lifestyle. Perhaps learning some great facts and ideas, may help you to create a plant based main dish along with a side of meat instead of the other way around.

I personally have taken my health to the next level and understand what it takes to be serious about avoiding disease and illness. When others see you practicing what you preach, they are inspired and want to learn how to make it happen for themselves. Because I am nearing my 60th birthday and have the education and experience, it has become my passion to become a Healthy Aging Expert. I have arrived. Nutrition is my expertise.

This book is long overdue. Over the last few years, life got in the way and my book was put on a shelf. Does this sound familiar? Many of us have "stuff" happen and then we allow it to slow down or halt our dreams and goals. 2013 was a pretty crazy year for me that led to putting it off even longer. Then about 6 months ago, one thing lead to another and to another and here we are. I woke up one day and decided that my book would be completed and published in early 2016. Period. No more excuses. Done.

Being in medicine well over 30+ years, I have seen the end result of when someone does not take their health seriously. I have seen the end result of the "could of, would of, should of's." I see people regret their past lifestyle and don't believe in themselves enough to make changes even in their 50's, 60's, 70's and older. I now know that if I can help inspire even one more person, then this journey will all be worth it.

What do I want my readers to get out of this book? I would like to put some serious life changing thoughts into my reader's mind. I would like to share my expertise and influence better health decisions and behaviors. What they do with the information is up to them. My goal is to share the lifestyle and nutrition knowledge I have. If I can help change our country's health direction for the positive, then I have done my job. Even if it's only one success story at a time.

Thoughts for my readers…

What if …you woke up tomorrow and received a serious diagnosis from your doctor? Then you are told that you may have avoided it had you been on a good plant based nutrition plan, decreased your stress and exercised more.

What if …you looked in the mirror and noticed how rapidly your skin changes have been? Then you realize that all you eat is processed food, drink tons of coffee and sleep on as little as 4 hours a night by choice.

What if …you ran into an old high school friend you haven't seen in 40 years and he or she did not even recognize you because of all the unhealthy weight you have gained? Then you realize that your excuse was that you have the "someday syndrome?" Someday I will lose the weight, someday I will get healthy, someday...

What if ...you died at 50 and when you went to heaven, you were told that your life would have been extended much longer had you quit smoking? That you literally have been pouring chemicals into your lungs with each and every puff.

What if ...you told yourself how hard it was to keep your blood sugars under control and therefore gave excuse after excuse to your doctor when your lab tests came back abnormal? Then what did it feel like when the doctor told you that your sight or kidneys were failing?

I strongly advise you NOT to live with the "someday syndrome" or the "what if's?" Make those words nonexistent in your daily thought. Make a decision. Make a strong and healthy one and then let me and others help you move forward.

Getting healthy and staying healthy from your local grocery store, farmers market, health food store or even your own garden may be hard for some people because of the lack of knowledge. There are groups of people that have grown up on "fast or convenience foods" only because that's all their parents knew. I love "fast and convenient" and believe me you can do that too with the right foods, right mindset and planning ahead.

There are numerous "diet plans" out there that literally feed you all your meals. People want that so they don't have to think or plan. Problem is, you don't know what to do when you cannot afford or are tired of those kinds of meals.

Let me share with you a true story…

Jason (name changed) was a 63-year-old patient that I met in 2010 when he walked into my office without an appointment and in tears. He asked for an appointment right away, so I worked him into my busy schedule that day. This man looked distraught and I knew he needed to talk.

Jason shared with me how much he weighed (360 lbs), and said that his weight was an issue for his entire life and obviously his health had really suffered from it. He was only 5' 9". Jason was now on several medications and was desperate. He had tried every kind of diet, giving up because the results weren't fast enough and he felt worse.

Jason also had a gastric lap band placed a few years ago, but then he self-taught himself how to get more food passed the band. In fact, he lost 80 lbs right after the procedure but unfortunately has gained back almost all of it. I asked Jason if he went to see a nutritionist before his surgery so that he could work through his food addictions. He told me that he "just had to attend a couple classes with a bunch of people in it."

Sadly, I've heard this from other patients so I knew he was not stretching or omitting the truth. People with weight issues can have a serious eating disorder, no matter what they weigh. We think of an eating disorder as anorexia or bulimia, not when someone is normal size or overweight. Being obese is a sign that your ability to feed your taste buds what it wants is strong and the ability to limit your intake and chose healthier foods is poor.

I asked Jason, why the tears? He explained to me that his three daughters were scared. They all lived out of town and have seen his struggle and wanted to help. They had already lost their mother (at age 48) to a "sudden death heart attack" only 2 years earlier and did not want the same thing to happen to their dad.

So they decided to get their dad into a program that would mail him his meals every month. Then all he needed to do was eat one for breakfast, lunch and dinner. Simple, or so they thought. The program offered nutritional guidance online and had all kinds of celebrity endorsements. But there was one problem. It was only January 11th and Jason admitted that he'd eaten ALL 90 of the meals sent to him. FYI: Placing 90 prepared food trays in front of someone with an eating disorder does NOT fix the disorder. Jason was sad and very remorseful that he did this and knew his daughters would be disappointed with him. They were the ones paying for all the meals.

I then asked Jason if he'd ever received 1:1 nutritional counseling for an extended period and he said no. I told him that this may be the biggest challenge of his life, but if he was willing to listen, learn and act on it that I would help him. We set up a time to call his daughters. In fact, the daughters were very forgiving (which put a smile on Jason's face) and they agreed to pay for my services because of their dad's limited income. Jason and I also called and cancelled the meal service that day.

I saw Jason for quite some time. Not only did I have private sessions with him but he attended every one of my cooking class that he could. Jason also received some biofeedback and hypnotherapy along with starting a walking group with his neighbors. As of July 2011, Jason lost well over 170 lbs!!! He did this without medications, diet pills or prepared meals (other than those he prepared himself). He learned how valuable eating a plant based diet was. Jason loved fish so over the course of the 18 months he eventually became a Pescetarian (a vegetarian that includes fish into their plant based diet). Jason learned to create meals that were full of nutrients, minerals and so much more. He not only lost the weight but was completely off of all his prescribed medications.

Jason's success story took A LOT of hard work, tears, smiles and education that he was willing to commit to. Since then he has relocated with his family to the east coast and continues to do well.

To all of the Jason's in the world, I want you to know that there is help out there and realize that it may not be easy. You may fail several times. But it's ok. It's the end result you are after. Remember, NOTHING rocks successful weight loss like increasing your knowledge of good nutrition and exercise then following through. There is no short cut.

"Health is the soul that animates

all the enjoyments of life,

which fade and are tasteless

without it."

~ Lucius Annaeus Seneca

Chapter 3

The Impact of Good Nutrition on Disease

What we do today will follow us tomorrow. Want healthy skin? Healthy internal organs? Energy? Weight loss? Most of us want it all – but are not willing to do whatever it takes to reach those results.

Disease is defined a few ways according to the dictionary:

1. A disordered or incorrectly functioning organ, part, structure, or system of the body resulting from the effect of genetic or developmental errors, infection, poisons, nutritional deficiency or imbalance, toxicity, or unfavorable environmental factors; illness; sickness; ailment.

2. Any abnormal condition in a plant that interferes with its vital physiological processes, caused by pathogenic, microorganisms, parasites, unfavorable environmental, genetic, or nutritional factors, etc.

3. Any harmful, depraved, or morbid condition, as of the mind or society.

4. Decomposition of a material under special circumstances.

5. To affect with disease; make ill.

The human body needs certain nutrients on a daily basis to fight illness/disease and to maintain homeostasis where the body stays in balance. A body in balance can avoid many issues. Having a great immune system in itself is vital to every age. Studies have shown that the average American who consumes a plant based diet, one with whole foods like vegetables, fruits, grains and legumes have proven to have a much lower incidence of chronic diseases especially as they age.

Sadly, in America, our diets still continue to be surrounded by highly processed foods, saturated fats and trans fats. Sugars from corn (high fructose corn sugars) are rampant in our grocery stores, therefore, they end up in many grocery carts and carried into our homes. This type of diet along with a sedentary lifestyle has led to unprecedented amounts of heart disease, cancers, Type II diabetes and a long list of other illnesses that many researchers now say could be avoided with a plant based diet.

We are what we eat. No doubt. "Let food be thy medicine" has been preached by the smartest in the world for centuries. A strong plant based diet can maintain health along with prevent disease. So when I came up with the motto for my company: "Eat the Way YOU Want to Look", I wanted others to realize that what goes into our guts, our engines, is what you see on the outside showing through your energy, vitality, your skin and then internally in every cell. What you eat, how much you eat is vital to how each and every cell works on a moment to moment basis.

Cancers are closely studied and it has been found that some have direct correlation to our diets and our excess weight. Sugar has a direct impact on healing, on wellness and prevention of serious life threatening diseases. Obesity has affected every aspect of our public health system and with no obvious end in sight, it makes you wonder where the world will be in another 10 years if we are not able to make a dent in it.

Today, we literally have hundreds of medical professionals like Dr. Oz who have made it their passion to help change the way Americans look at their food, their health and to really understand the impact it has on each other. I love that he teaches on his show. He has impacted and saved more lives than he will never know. Watching his show is one thing, listening, really listening to him can start to change your life.

Listen, then act, following through.

Listen, then act, following through.

Rinse and repeat.

Healthy eating is only hard if you

tell yourself that it is.

"I've made a promise to myself

to be

a 100% healthier person

if nothing else."

~ Picabo Street

"Being in control of your life and

having realistic

expectations about your day-to-day

challenges are the

keys to stress management,

which is perhaps the most important

ingredient to living a

happy, healthy and rewarding life."

~ Marilu Henner

Chapter 4

My Path to Becoming a Nutrition & Health Expert

My education started out in the nursing field in the 1970's. My desire to help others has been with me since I was in my early teens. After I graduated from high school, I became an RN and worked in an array of different medical and nursing industries. My passion was not only to take care of my patients but to teach them how to improve and manage their own health, avoiding future issues and live life with intention.

Living well, I would say, is everyone's desire. Doing what it takes to get there is a different topic. But I feel that without the education and support, they don't know how to change.

In the early days of my career, I always felt like the "nutrition component" was missing big time. I would see my patients fight for their health and yet the medical facilities they were staying at would feed them diets of overcooked vegetables, processed meats, instant mashed potatoes, white rolls and deserts made with high sugar and fat. Unless the patient was on a specific diet (i.e. diabetic) and then I felt like those menus may have met the calorie count but not always the nutritional need.

Over the years, I have had dietician friends who had to follow the government standards that they were taught even if they did not always agree. We've known for years the impact that certain foods have on our bodies along with the ability to heal and perhaps prevent many illnesses. Food definitely impacts health, no doubt.

I decided to extensively increase my education with as much nutritional knowledge as possible. People need to heal and when we solve their immediate health problems and then return them home without making a dietary impact, all we are doing is creating a ricochet effect. Today, I will admit that many medical facilities are improving the types of meals being served. Kudos to them!

I realized decades ago that knowledge is power. Does that mean that every patient listens to and follows your instructions? No, I wish. However, you have to give the patient the knowledge and have follow up available to them. Hospital stays are much shorter and each discipline has so much to share with each patient as they literally whisk them out the door. But then what happens to these discharged patients?

There were 3 things I felt were missing from patient care. (1) An increase in "plant based nutrition" incorporated into the diets (2) Stress management techniques taught because it absolutely did effect their health (3) Life skills to manage their future and current health issues. Primary practitioners should fill in that gap referring their patients to a variety of professional resources. Unfortunately, it doesn't always happen. Could it be that they are overbooked with patients and short on time or perhaps they have no idea what to do or where to send them? Some medical practitioners do a phenomenal job of getting their patients the help they need.

Bottom line, we need to look past the disease and focus on the kind of wellness our nation needs. Obesity has become acceptable and is driving our health care costs up. A holistic team approach is actually starting to become the norm in certain areas of our country, which is fantastic.

Increasing my education was a passion I followed through on. I believed that if I knew more, I could help more people. So I became Certified in Nutrition, Stress Management and became a Professional Life Coach. Then as a Certified Holistic Practitioner I learned to combine eastern and western medicine with success. It took more time and energy but I love what I do. Then almost 10 years ago, I became a professional speaker who loves to teach and motivate. Blending all of my education together has really created the perfect career for me to help a wide range of individuals.

Several years ago, I was blessed to start my own medical practice and received referrals from all over the country. I founded Balanced Health 101 and The Self Improvement Center in Southern New Mexico. Inside the walls of my business, I offered many holistic services that was recommended for my patients. Nutrition, Massage, Biofeedback, Hypnotherapy, Tai Chi, Meditation and Yoga was provided by highly trained practitioners. It was a very successful practice with thousands of patients.

Then in 2012, I closed my practice and decided to take my skills on the road. Since then I have grown my professional speaking and seminar business "Influential Success", teaching and inspiring every one along the way. I speak on a very wide array of topics and again, love what I do. Whether speaking to just 10 or 100 or literally 1000's at a time, it has been an amazing ride! Life is good.

"A healthy outside starts

from the inside."

~ Robert Urich

Chapter 5

Eating for Longevity

What is the difference between "eating for longevity" or "eating for survival"? Eating for survival will get you from day to day. Eating for longevity will not only change your energy levels, it will affect the way your skin looks, how your internal organs function and will slow down the aging process. What a difference a healthy lifestyle makes compared to a poor lifestyle. Which do you prefer?

Interesting statistics on the "Standard American Diet" (according to Wikipedia).

The "Standard American Diet" (S.A.D.) is a similar term, specifically used to describe the stereotypical diet of Americans. The typical American diet is about 50% carbohydrate, 15% protein, and 35% fat, [5] which is over the dietary guidelines for the amount of fat (below 30%), below the guidelines for carbohydrate (above 55%), and at the upper end of the guidelines for the amount of protein (below 15%) recommended in the diet.

The quality of the carbohydrate, protein, and fat is at least as important as the quantity. Complex carbohydrates such as starch are believed to be healthier than the sugar so frequently consumed in the Standard American Diet.

The Standard American Diet is high in saturated fat, but it is estimated that for every 1% of saturated fat energy that is replaced with polyunsaturated fat there would be more than a 2-3% reduction in coronary heart disease incidence. And even for polyunsaturated fat, the high levels of omega-6 fatty acids compared to omega-3 fatty acids in the Western diet is believed to contribute to autoimmune and inflammatory diseases as well as cancer and cardiovascular disease.

A review of eating habits in the United States in 2004 found that about 75% of restaurant meals were from fast-food restaurants, whereas only 1% were fine food dining restaurants. Nearly half of the meals ordered from a menu were hamburger, French fries, or poultry — and about one third of orders included a carbonated beverage drink. From 1970 to 2008, the per capita consumption of calories increased by nearly one-quarter in the United States and about 10% of all calories were from high-fructose corn syrup.

Health concerns

Compared to the "prudent" diet, the Western pattern diet, based on epidemiological studies of Westerners, is positively correlated with an elevated incidence of obesity, death from heart disease, cancer (especially colon cancer), and other "Western pattern diet"-related diseases. Breast cancer epidemiologists have identified a "Western/Unhealthy" dietary pattern that is high in red/processed meats, refined grains, potatoes, *sweets, and high-fat dairy by means of multivariate statistics methods, like principal components analysis and factor analysis; they find that, overall, women with a more Western diet have an increased risk of breast cancer that is not statistically significant.*

Wow. Look around and understand that if we are to change and become more of a "preventative society" instead of a "treatment society", then we need to reverse this unhealthy way of eating. Knowledge along with the desire to improve the Standard American Diet (SAD) can and will change obesity statistics. Then we can lower incidences of diseases that are related to poor nutrition, lack of exercise and high stress. Consuming a diet high in complex carbohydrates, one that is plant-based and high in fiber would result in a lower incidence of cancer and coronary artery disease along with dozens of others.

"Take care of your body,

it's the only place you have to live."

~ Jim Rohn

Chapter 6

Your Body's Warranty
Filling Your
Engine with Powerful Foods

I noticed several years ago, that many people took better care of their vehicles than they did their own bodies. They take their cars in for oil changes, perhaps put in a higher quality gas, if they hear the slightest ping or irregular sound they run it in to the shop. If the engine light comes on they act on it, when it reaches certain miles they follow the maintenance schedule, they wash it, they show it off, then they panic if something happens and the car is out of warranty. Why does this happen? Because they paid a lot of $$$ for their vehicle and it may cost them more if they neglect routine checkups and needed maintenance. Interestingly, the average car last 8-10 years and YOU CAN REPLACE IT as needed throughout your lifetime.

Now let's look at our bodies. Many people ONLY go to the doctor when their "pings" or "symptoms" become very obvious. They put "bad gas and oil" into their ENGINES every day with poor eating habits, consuming many processed foods and GMO's that are ladened with chemicals and preservatives. They spend a fortune on making their bodies look good on the outside with expensive lotions and potions, yet what they eat affects their outer shell much more than they can ever imagine. We have NO warranty so "routine maintenance" is vital for longevity. Let me ask you, how much is YOUR body worth? Currently the average human being lives 70-80 years. We only get one body and YOU CANNOT REPLACE IT in your lifetime.

In my practice, I saw a variety of health issues. I was really amazed at how many people had the start of serious issues and did not make an appointment until it scared them. I took referrals from all over the country and one thing was consistent. Very few people came to see me when they were feeling well and just wanted to be sure they were doing everything possible to stay that way.

For decades in this country, we are taught to go to our health care professional when we have an issue instead of planning a "well visit" just to see what can be done at this stage in your life for prevention. The costs are remarkably less along with the suffering and taxing financial issues when an illness is found and the need for expensive medical treatments begin.

"When you are young and healthy,

it never occurs to you

that in a single second

your whole life could change."

~ Annette Funicello

Chapter 7

Procrastination and Your Health

For those of you reading this book and perhaps looking for answers or inspiration, let me share my thoughts on procrastination when it comes to your health and eating well. *What we do to our bodies today, we will pay for tomorrow.*

Why do so many people start taking care of themselves or take better care of themselves AFTER a life changing illness occurs? Going to the doctor when we are sick is expected, however, I have had patients who delayed going when they should of and suffered serious consequences for the delay.

Over the past 50+ years, America had become more of a "treatment based" health care system than a "preventative" one. I believe it is starting to change and for medical professionals like myself, we are pushing prevention more than ever. An increased number of businesses are looking at the health of their employees and realizing that it can and does affect their insurance costs, sick time and productivity. A healthy employee can be a huge asset, while an employee with current health problems and no desire to change can affect their overall bottom line. Unfortunately, high insurance deductibles and the cost of health care deters many from seeing their health care provider on a regular basis.

Then there are those with "symptoms" that live with this belief "if I don't know what's wrong and there is no diagnosis yet – then it must not exist." So they avoid seeing a practitioner until their symptoms are getting in the way of life. If you think this way, you are a time bomb waiting to explode. Prevention along with early detection would be your absolute very best health plan.

Let me share a study I did in 2011, in our southern NM town of approximately 38k residents. I wondered how many individuals had made some significant improvements in their daily health habits over the past year and what happened to move them in that direction?

I interviewed well over 100 walkers. Several of them I already knew in our community, along with dozens that Mall walked in the early am and others pacing themselves along the Scenic Drive walking path next to the mountains. I asked 3 questions. First, how long have you been walking? Next, what prompted you to start? Last, how is your health? What I learned, had opened my eyes to how many people ONLY took action because of 2 main reasons. First, weight loss was a biggie but the number two reason was they either had a health scare or major health event. I heard everything from: heart attack, diabetes, cholesterol issues, stroke or an obesity related illnesses (which there are many including some types of cancers.) ONLY about a dozen of the participants were actually doing it to "prevent" disease and had no trace of medical issues currently.

Do YOU need a wakeup call?

You may have "SOMEDAY SYNDROME". Someday - I will start walking. Someday - I will lose this weight. Someday - I will control my blood sugars. Someday - I will take better care of me. Someday...ugh. Face the music and do what you know you need to do.

What we do to our bodies today, we will pay for tomorrow. There are diseases that can be reversed with good nutrition, exercise and decreasing the amount of stress in your life. On the other side of the coin, there are numerous conditions and diseases that harm your body along the way, and repairing the damages becomes the center of your focus. Being ill can cause financial burdens on you and your family. It can cause a huge amount of emotional stress on relationships perhaps ending in divorce, depression and/or anxiety. You've seen it happen to others, it's overwhelmingly sad. Don't let it happen to you.

My challenge to you is, WHY WAIT? Stop the patterns in your life that will perhaps alter how you live (i.e. stroke) or cause an early death. Look at making small changes every day so that at the end of 6 months you have made some major strides towards a healthier future.

Hopefully, this book will be the start of you taking a long hard look at your habits, health status and family history. Then you can really work on prevention more than expensive and life altering treatments.

"I believe that the greatest gift

you can give your family

and the world is a

healthier you."

~ Joyce Meyer

Chapter 8

Aging, Cancer and Sugar

As we age, exposures in our diets, chemicals and poor lifestyles increase our risk for cancer. Excessive sugar intake in the American diets have increase every decade. There truly is a sugar addiction in our country. Sugar is added to many products that you would never expect. It's also a major inflammatory food that can promote abnormal growths within our bodies. So as you age, avoiding as much sugar as possible will give you a much better chance of aging well and avoiding disease.

Here are some negative effects that sugar can have:

• Sugar promotes belly fat. Mix that with hormonal changes and your fighting that menopausal/sugar muffin top. Ugh, who wants that?

• Sugar can damage your heart by increasing your risk for health disease. One study showed strong evidence that sugar can actually affect the pumping mechanism of your heart. When this happens you increase your chances for heart failure.

• Too much sugar can be toxic to your liver. Our liver is the organ that filters everything that goes through our circulatory systems. When you clog your liver, it is like clogging the engine in your car. Boom. It's not going anywhere.

• Here is an eye opener as we age. There was a study that found a relationship between glucose consumption and the aging of our cells. From wrinkles to chronic disease. Another alarming study showed that excess sugar may affect the aging of your brain. Excess sugar consumption has been linked to deficiencies in memory and cognitive health. Not sure about you – but I limit any sugar I can. Too much strong research involving the demise of our brains on sugar. I want to avoid those diseases if at all possible!

• Sugar, especially in excess, may be linked to some cancers and may limit cancer survival. Again, sugar inflammation can cause rhetoric in our bodies.

There was an article written in Shape Magazine online called "Does Sugar Really Cause Cancer?" The studies they wrote about came from very reputable resources and is worth reading.

These are few of the highlights:

- A new study published in Cancer Research suggests that you might want to add sugar to the list of cancer causing agents.
- Researchers at the University of Texas MD Anderson Cancer Center fed infant mice

(genetically pre-disposed to breast cancer) either low-sugar, starchy diets or high-sugar ones. Then, researchers looked at them at six months old. Of the mice that had eaten levels of sugar similar to those found in the average American diet, 60 percent had breast cancer. On the other hand, only 30 percent of mice on a low-sugar diet had breast cancer. What's more, breast cancer tumors were larger, grew more quickly, and had more often spread to the lungs in the sugar-loaded mice.

- The study also found that fructose, a simple sugar molecule contained in table sugar and high-fructose corn syrup, increased the body's expression of proteins and fatty acids that contribute to cancer growth.
- "The take-home message is that everyone, particularly those who are at a high risk of cancer or already have cancer, should reduce their added sugar intake from processed foods, table sugar, and sugar-sweetened beverages," says Peiying Yang, Ph.D., an assistant professor of palliative, rehabilitation, and integrative medicine at MD Anderson, and co-author of the study.
- In 2012, a study from the National Cancer Institute, researchers followed 435,674 men and women for more than seven years and found that people who consumed more added sugar had higher rates of esophageal

adenocarcinoma, small intestine cancer, and cancer in the lining of the lungs.

Bottom line, if you have a pretty big sugar addiction, get help. Sugar in your life can add a wonderfully sweet taste to it once in a while, however, it's the daily and moderate use you may want to re-think.

To read the entire article go to:

http://www.shape.com/healthy-eating/does-sugar-really-cause-cancer

"To keep the body in good health

is a duty...

otherwise we shall not be able to keep

our mind strong and clear."

~ Buddha

Chapter 9

Artificial Sweeteners

&

The Aging Brain

My personal story of consuming excess amounts of artificial sweeteners started back in the early 70's while I was in high school. Tab was the "big diet soda." I really liked the flavor and I was one of those people who believed that if I saved a few calories here and there then I could maintain my weight and eat the extra foods that I liked. But it became a HUGE addiction for years, even decades.

Even back then I knew that it was not the best beverage of choice. I consumed very little water because in my mind, the soda had some water in it. Hmmm. What was I thinking??? I knew it may affect children/babies differently so I totally avoided any artificial sweeteners each and every time I was pregnant. I remember my last pregnancy, I craved it so much but never crossed the line. I knew that my baby (now 27 years old) needed to have the best environment to grow in and what if those chemicals got to her? I counted the days. Then when I was on my way to the hospital to give birth, I had my husband buy me a 6 pack. Even though I would not touch it till I finished breastfeeding her. I wanted it sitting there even if it was weeks/months till I could actually drink it. Nuts huh? No, diet soda addictions can be very real.

For years, everywhere I went I had my Tab or Fresca or Diet Coke with me. I even panicked when I would get down to a couple of cans at home, sort of like when an alcoholic thinks their stash is almost gone. It was ridiculous but real none the less.

Then I started to really study nutrition. I loved learning and it sparked something in me. I was learning so much that was not taught to me in my nursing school nutrition class. I started to learn about what different foods did to our bodies and how to really eat healthy.

One day I thought - could I ever give up diet soda? I knew with each can that I was filling my body with chemicals and it was not good for my health, or for my bones because of the phosphoric acid. Read a soda label, diet and regular, it's scary. Diet Coke has carbonated water, caramel color, aspartame, phosphoric acid, potassium citrate, natural flavors, citric acid, and caffeine. I tried on several occasions to decrease the amount I consumed to one can per day but would eventually go back to the 4-5 cans per day like before. I also thought, am I teaching my children well by drinking this stuff?

My education in nutrition continued, I became passionate about knowing as much as I could. I loved eating well and was excited when I could maintain my weight without being on any fad or unhealthy diet. But the one thing I was missing in my healthy life was more water and no diet soda. I also knew many doctors and other medical professionals including dieticians that drank the stuff too – so that was another added excuse in my mind and I put the decision off for years.

Then in 2002, I woke up one day and looked in the mirror and said to myself, "enough is enough." I am filling my body with chemicals while trying to inspire others to eat well. Crazy. We were going on a boat trip that day, our coolers were full of great healthy snacks along with a nutrition packed lunch – and of course diet drinks. While we were on the boat I looked at my family and said, "today is the last day you will see me drink any Diet Coke or Tab." I remembered them thinking it wasn't going to happen and my husband said "yeah" (kind of like - yeah, right). I could not believe that they did not think I was serious!! Not only do I keep my promises to my family but their doubts caused me stop this crazy addiction even more. I knew that doing it "cold turkey" and announcing it to my family would be the best way for me to quit 100%. I drank my last Diet Coke in July 2002 in T or C, New Mexico. It may not seem like a big deal to many of you, but for those addicted to diet soda, you understand.

The results were huge. First, anytime you can successfully give up an unhealthy food addiction, whether to diet soda, regular soda, sugar, processed foods, chips, cookies, ice cream, etc. it is an accomplishment. Diet soda as an occasional drink is not a major issue. Neither is a cookie or ice cream. But consuming unhealthy foods daily or several times per week can affect your long term health.

I was excited, my skin improved greatly. I slept better. My cravings for processed foods literally dissolved about a month later because I wasn't fooling my brain any longer. I was ecstatic and healthy.

What do I drink for fluids these days?

I taught myself to find the healthiest drinks possible and then learn to love them or at least like them. Water became my very best friend. I love tea...hot or cold, green or black, absolutely plain with NO sweetener. I drink fresh organic lemon water every morning. I also love fruit or veggie infused water and enjoy a cup of delicious black organic coffee. I drink nothing with sweeteners or additives. Boring perhaps, but my long term health and skin are much more important as I age. Remember my motto "Eat (or drink) the way YOU want to look."

So as I share the rest of this chapter, really look at your health and how YOU want to age. Realize that "artificial anything" does not help you age well. What was hard for me for years, may be easy for you to stop or slow down. No matter what you get out of this book, make a decision TODAY to lessen your chemical exposure and increase your antioxidants and exercise for a long and healthy lifestyle!!!

"Can I switch to artificial sweeteners to save calories and be safe?" This was a commonly asked question from my patients.

Artificial sweeteners (AS) are a HUGE industry in America, millions perhaps billions of dollars are made off of individuals who wanted to save a few calories or diabetics who needed to have less of a sugar spike and turned to the multitudes of sweeteners that are artificially made.

The AS manufacturers state that they are considered safe in low to moderate amounts. Practitioners, nutritionists, dieticians and others who have degrees and/or much knowledge in human nutrition, argue otherwise. Studies have been done on lab rats and it has been concluded that yes, AS can affect us in a negative way. However, we are not rats – but I also do not want to be a human testing ground.

Reading labels to see what kind of AS is in any product can sometimes take a scientist or chemist to understand it exactly. The history of AS started with saccharin in the late 1800's. It was discovered by a lab chemist who was working with coal tar. Coal tar, if you don't know, is a carcinogenic material. Hmmm, don't know about you but it's discovery does not sit well with something I want to ingest into my body frequently, or ever, if I can avoid it.

There are actually 5 artificial sweeteners approved and sold in America.

- Saccharin (may be labeled as sodium saccharin, calcium saccharin or acid saccharin) Its sweetness level is 300 times sweeter than sugar. Sweet 'N Low (pink packet) is a common AS that you would recognize the most, along with Necta Sweet.

- Aspartame (may be labeled as dextrose w/ maltodextrin aspartame) Its sweetness is approximately 180 times sweeter than sugar. NutraSweet (the blue packets) and Equal are the most common names you will see. When aspartame enters your body, it breaks into 2 amino acids: aspartic acid and phenylalanine along with a small amount of wood alcohol. Aspartame *should not* be used to cook with because it is not stable at cooking and baking temperatures. Aspartic acid in aspartame is a well-studied and documented excitotoxin. Excitotoxins can cause a loss of brain synapses along with connecting fibers. There is so much to read about excitotoxins online. Just know that anything that causes loss of brain synapses I assure you - will NOT be a part of my healthy aging lifestyle.

- Acesulfame K (may be labeled as acesulfame potassium) is approximately 200 times sweeter than sugar and cannot be metabolized by the body. Sunett along with Sweet One are the most common you will find (there are others). It is used in dry beverages, dairy products, candy, chewing gum, dessert mixes, alcoholic beverages, chocolate confections, baked goods and carbonated drinks.

- Neotame is the baby of AS and is 40 times sweeter than aspartame, however, thousands (7-8k) sweeter than sugar. It is composed of aspartic acid and phenylalanine. Neotame is used as a table top sweetener. It can also be used in some of the same foods/beverages as acesulfame K and aspartame.

- Sucralose (may be labeled as dextrose, maltodextrin and sucralose) It is 600 times sweeter than sugar and is the most heat stable AS, so you will see it added to many baked items. Sucralose started as sucrose and by a chemist changing its molecular structure they developed it into this AS. It is only about 16 years old and sold as Splenda (yellow packet.)

What do Artificial Sweeteners do to our bodies and minds that have caused concern?

As we age, our hormones go thru a multitude of changes, some good and some not. Keeping our bodies in a "positive hormonal homeostasis" is important to feeling good, looking good and being healthy.

Artificial sweeteners literally mess with your hormones, especially insulin. When you taste anything sweet your body releases insulin (even if it had no calories) as if you'd eaten real sugar. Of course we know that the release of insulin leads to blood sugars issues and that can and does increase cravings. Initially, people are trying to avoid calories and they end up craving more high caloric foods, which if consumed, can increase your weight. AS can literally have the opposite effect of what your reason for consuming them were. There is nothing more irritating as you age when you gain weight in the abdominal area (as a possible side effect of AS added into your diet.)

Because they are so sweet, they expose your taste buds to higher levels of it. Now, you may not enjoy that simple piece of fruit or you will want to keep adding more sweetener to your foods or you may seek out higher caloric sweet foods resulting in weight gain and other metabolic issues. Keeping your taste buds intact as you age is important to enjoy delicious foods for years to come.

Another issue with AS is that they are genetically modified. Many of them are made from GMO sugar beets, corn or soy. My stance on GMO (genetically modified) foods is to omit as many of them in your diet as possible. I believe that current studies have given us much reason to avoid them. Again, I am not looking to personally become a "study rat" and find out years later that the current findings were 100% correct.

AS also increases the risk of diabetes. Researchers aren't clear if biological changes are happening because of the AS or whether people consume other unhealthy or high caloric foods with it. Perhaps they feel that they are "saving calories" in one area so they over eat in other areas. It is estimated that 60-70% of people who consumed diet sodas were most likely overweight. The increase in Type II diabetics in the past decade in America is statistically alarming. It has become a very common health challenge and has driven health care costs up along with financial and emotional tolls on families and caregivers.

In the early 70's when I was in high school, children had Type I Diabetes (an autoimmune disease unrelated to diet.) Today, Type II has become a major health challenge for children too. How sad. Back then adults had Type II but NOT in the *masses we see today.*

What has changed over the past 40 years? It is a huge cause for concern and one we can start to learn from. Our food industry is growing at a rapid pace and "convenience" is the "Name of The Grocery Game." Hidden sugars (AS and cane sugars) are used as fillers and sweeteners.

Reading labels are vital just to understand what you are purchasing and feeding your family. Caloric dense snacks are cheap and easy to buy at any store, gas station and sadly even in some hospital vending machines.

You may wonder, what kind of safe natural sweeteners are there?

Stevia comes from a plant and is not artificial. It is safe for diabetics. Stevia is quite popular these days and manufacturers are trying to replace it in many products because of its popularity. Many nutritionists use it on several different types of foods. I suggest, as with all sweeteners, use it sparingly. Plus, it is a little bitter when you use too much.

Others natural sweeteners that people may use:

Honey

Agave Nectar

Raw, unprocessed sugar

Brown Rice Syrup

Barley Malt

Maple Syrup

Xylitol

Things I personally do to sweetened dishes. I use fresh squeezed fruit juice like mango directly on my salads. Unsweetened applesauce in place of oils and to add a sweet taste for my homemade breads (banana, pumpkin, etc.) I drizzle maple syrup lightly over dishes that may need a little sweetness to them. Just like artificial sweeteners, once you get away from that taste and start to enjoy real live foods surprisingly your taste buds will change and your health will become even stronger. Remember, too many sweets produce consistent inflammation within your body and can set you up for possible health issues. Healthy aging is all about decreasing the inflammation!

So as I wrap up this chapter, I want you to understand that we all have to protect our health because *we only have one go around.* Having this knowledge put things into perspective for me years ago. Now that you know more about artificial sweeteners, perhaps you will pay closer attention to reading labels, or limit the amount of chemicals and additives in your foods OR most importantly your children's foods. *To live a long healthy life, you must put what you know into practice.*

"The winners in life treat their body as if

it was a magnificent spacecraft

that gives them the finest transportation

and endurance for their lives."

~ Denis Waitley

Chapter 10

Metabolic Syndrome
Becoming a Commonly Used
Diagnosis in Medicine

WebMD states that...

"Metabolic syndrome is a health condition that everyone's talking about."

"Although it was only identified less than 20 years ago, metabolic syndrome is as widespread as pimples and the common cold. According to the American Heart Association, 47 million Americans have it. That's almost a staggering one out of every six people. The syndrome runs in families and is more common among African-Americans, Hispanics, Asians, and Native Americans. The risks of developing metabolic syndrome increases as you age."

"Metabolic syndrome is not a disease in itself. Instead, it's a group of risk factors -- high blood pressure, high blood sugar, unhealthy cholesterol levels, and abdominal fat."

"Obviously, having any one of these risk factors isn't good. But when they're combined, they set the stage for serious problems. These risk factors double your risk of blood vessel and heart disease, which can lead to heart attacks and strokes. They increase your risk of diabetes by five times."

They say that "the good news is that metabolic syndrome can be controlled, largely with changes to your lifestyle."

Why has this happened?

These are some of the reasons I see metabolic syndrome becoming such a common (but scary and growing) diagnosis:

• The sedentary lifestyles many individuals have developed. No longer are we working in the fields or tending to our farms like decades ago. We have jobs that entail sitting at computers or technology. We are not as physical as our ancestors and it's catching up to us.

• Exercise is not a huge part of our daily living. Gyms memberships are up but attendance is down. We join to make ourselves feel like we are doing something, but sticking to a routine becomes too inconvenient. We should strive for at least 30-60 minutes of exercise EVERY day. Recent studies have shown that if you are over 50 years old, more exercise is not necessarily better. Focus on cardio every day with weights 3-4 times per week. I prefer the treadmill so I can really challenge myself with speeds and the incline, then use exercise bands and weights of different sizes. Not only will that help my muscles but my bones as well.

• Sleep is a MAJOR answer to slowing down the aging process. Getting 7-8 hours a night of good sleep recharges your entire body and mind. Sleep deprivation can and will affect your health. You will see it in your skin, in your energy levels and your immune system can start to break down allowing a host of illnesses to happen. If, what I just described is you, get help finding out why you are not sleeping and if you already know the reason, then get help fixing it. Want to know what ages you fast – UNTREATED sleep apnea. It can cause inflammatory events within your body and may set you up for a possible heart attack or stroke while asleep. Bottom line, adequate sleep is HUGE for our brains along with healthy aging.

• The food and restaurant industry has changed. More "all you can eat buffets", more "super-sized or biggie meals" are popping up. "For only 50 cents more you can get twice as much fries." Of course you do not need them, but what the heck it's a deal.   Hmmm... dietary inflammation is preventable, it's just a decision away.

• The outside isles in our grocery stores usually have the healthier products. The inner isles are huge and full of quick, convenient and sugar/sodium filled products. Learning to cook from scratch is happening less and less. There are a lot of great recipes that take less than 30 minutes to prepare that would be a much healthier option for our families. People say they don't have time to cook every night. I read an article that says the average person who goes out or drives through routinely for their dinner (3-7 times per week) has a larger waistline, more belly fat, not so good cholesterol and by the time they get to the restaurant and order, 30-45 minutes have passed by anyway. How is that a time saver? Hmmm...

• Last but not least, STRESS. Our world is full of it and it's our jobs to find a way to not only decrease it, but more importantly decrease what it does to us. Our reactions are everything. The fight or flight response in stress increases chemicals within your body which then ages you. Cortisol can save lives when needed but it can also cause internal damage when the body suffers consistent stress. More doctor visits in the US are tied to stress more than any other reason. Stress can and will continue to kill people we love.

Want a great "healthy aging tip"? Find a way to decrease the stressors in your life.

Symptoms of elevated cortisol levels:

- You seem to gain weight quite easily even if you are eating well, exercising and trying to do everything possible. It tends to end up on your abdomen which can be frustrating.
- You easily catch every bug around (or it seems that way). Cortisol deactivates the job of the immune system which make you a target for viruses.
- You have a difficult time sleeping well even when you are tired. Regardless if you think

you slept ok, you can feel exhausted the next day.

- Sex isn't even a thought, or a passing one. Stress hormones from a high cortisol level decreases your sex hormone. Then there is no interest.
- You just don't feel happy at all because of the lack of serotonin in your body from the stress.
- You have a bigger appetite for unhealthy foods because your insulin levels are erratic, causing you to crave certain foods.
- You feel edgy, anxious, panicky.
- Your whole internal system is out of sorts, causing gastrointestinal issues and headaches. High cortisol levels can really mess with our other hormones throwing us way off balance.

Any of these symptoms sound familiar?

My suggestion is whenever you visit your health care practitioner, bring a written list of all your symptoms or concerns so that she/he can piece the puzzle together. Whether it's metabolic syndrome, diabetes or high cortisol levels, getting your body back into balance is crucial for healthy aging and living a good life.

Need help with stress? I suggest a good therapist or life coach to help you sort through your days and figure out what is causing the stress and then how to avoid or lessen it. The time to get help is not when you are in the emergency room with a heart attack or other urgent illness.

Being totally stress free may not be 100% possible as we live in fast times, we work hard and have busy lives, however, living a life with as low of stress as possible should be your ultimate goal. It really is how you react to situations that drive your cortisol levels. As we age, we tend to become more laid back, past experiences in life help us to accept more things we cannot change.

I find that journaling and meditating daily along with an exercise program and eating healthy decreases my stress level a lot. I have learned to say no and also learned to avoid or limit exposure to people who are not adding a positive influence into my life. Taking care of inflammation from high cortisol levels is vital. Do whatever you must to make that happen.

"Someone has to stand up and

say the answer is

NOT another pill.

The answer is spinach."

~ Bill Maher

Chapter 11

9 Interesting Facts About
Fruits & Veggies

Fruits & Veggies are healthy in every form. Fresh is great but know that frozen can be just as nutritious as it is usually taken off the vine, etc. and frozen right away. Many grocery stores can be selling items that are "fresh" but picked a couple weeks ago. Frozen really rocks especially for berries and green veggies, which you should be consuming a little of everyday. If you buy canned be sure to check the label and chose a can that is not BPA (chemically) lined. As time goes on, companies are realizing that consumers are looking for BPA free containers. I love that the masses of consumers in our country have the ability (through choosing the right food items) to steer the direction of what is produced or manufactured.

So I suggest eating fresh, frozen, or even drink it in a smoothie and you'll get the same benefits! Do keep in mind that if you drink it, it has to be 100% juice, skin and all or completely blended in a smoothie like I do with my NutriBullet every morning. Brands with only 5-10% juice is obviously not going to be more nutritious and can have chemicals and dyes added to them.

Supporting your local farmer's market is always a way to get fresh fruits and veggies. Remember that just because it is bought from a local market does not mean "organic" unless specified - so be sure to wash properly. Toxins can still exist and cleaning is important. Washing fresh produce is mandatory to rid them of chemicals, bug leftovers, dirt, etc. Local markets not only inspire you to buy fresh but gives you a sense of giving back to your community of growers who care.

Fiber is a big deal and knowing the benefits is huge. It can help lower your cholesterol, regulate your blood sugar, create a fullness in your gut which can help with weight control and regulates your bowel movements. Cancer of the bowels can start long before you have symptoms. Keeping your system going on a regular basis will decrease your chances of possible bowel disease.

Ever heard – an apple a day keeps the doctor away? Apples are full of healthy nutrition except for the seeds which contain a small amount of cyanide. Important to know if you give your little ones an apple to snack on, let them know to only eat down to the core or even better just remove the seeds ahead of time.

Mushrooms are one of the highest antioxidant foods there is! Because of this, mushrooms really stimulate your immune system and go into overdrive creating a healthy state internally. In oriental medicine, the mushroom is priceless when it comes to treating multiple health issues. One serving per day of mushrooms provides almost a quarter of an adult's requirements of selenium. There is such a variety of mushrooms to try. Incorporating them into soups, stems, and a multitude of dishes as much as possible is recommended. They are definitely a superfood!

Grapefruits are among the most nutritious Vitamin C fruits out there. If you are currently on certain medications, my advice is to check with your pharmacist or medical provider to find out if consuming grapefruit could interfere with the medications that you are on. Many people think it's only if you take a statin that you need to stay away from grapefruit and that is not correct. There are other medications that are affected by consuming grapefruit. If concerned, call and ask your pharmacist, he/she will advise. However, if you are taking NO medications, I would include this amazing fruit in your diet as studies have shown that it can help with weight control and cancer prevention. Also, if your doctor or pharmacist says it's ok to eat with your current medications – definitely include it in your diet!

Did you know that tomatoes were originally considered a fruit? How did that happen? The reason tomatoes are actually considered a fruit because they have seeds. Then in the late 1800's, our government ruled that tomatoes were a vegetable. Back then they were traded and imported vegetables were taxed but not the imported fruits. Tomatoes were ruled as a vegetable so they could be taxed when entering into the US. Tomatoes are botanically a fruit but in the US they are legally a vegetable. Craziness happens with governmental money/taxes and our food.

The skin has the most nutrients. I stopped peeling my fruits and veggies unless the outside was not edible. My carrots, cucumbers and beets I put into my daily smoothie have been washed well but not peeled. I am consuming ALL of the nutrients. The nutrition is stored in the skin and removing the edible outside does not give you as many nutrients. I believe you may be wasting your nutrient dollars by peeling many of them. Not sure what skins you can eat? There are several so I would google it and go from there. I even grate my orange and lemon peels into different healthy dishes. Bottom line, if it's edible, include it in your "healthy aging basket."

Onions and garlic have healing properties and should be a part of your everyday meals if possible. They are both tremendously healthy containing sulfide compounds that help prevent many types of cancers. Leeks, scallions, chives and garlic are all related and have a variety of health benefits that are worth eating quite often. I definitely look for recipes that can include even a small amount. With nutrition, every little bit can make a huge difference.

According to the Natural Resources Defense Council: "American shoppers are collectively responsible for more wasted food than farmers, grocery stores, or any other part of the food-supply chain." "The average family spends a shocking $2,225 every year on *food they don't eat.* This problem is so massive that if food waste were a country, it would have the third-largest environmental footprint after the United States and China."

Sad. Shocking. My thoughts were, with today's budgets the average American cannot afford to waste almost $200 per month in food. Can you imagine if everyone really paid attention and did not waste that $2,225 per year? Could they use the extra $$ to purchase organic foods or perhaps go towards a vacation, or education, or give to a charity of their choice? They could also use the extra $$$ to help feed those less fortunate or just be able to save it for an emergency. I read some reports where the number was even higher. WOW. Let's not only look at our personal health but the health of our pocketbooks and our future food industry. Do food companies dangle too much or do we over estimate the amount of food our families can consume? Whichever it is, take good a look at your household and make a conscious decision.

"Investing in health

will produce

enormous benefits."

~ Gro Harlem Brundhand

Chapter 12

Is Eating Healthy
More Expensive?

It's been said by many people that "it's too expensive to eat healthy." Bottom line - being unhealthy and being ill, is NOT cheap. But until you are faced with that reality, you may not understand. When you compare potato chips to whole potatoes, the whole potato is cheaper per pound. Convenience along with food addictions has widened our waistlines and made it easier to buy poor nutrients than the better choices.

I want you to know that I do understand budgets, we certainly learned how to really stretch the dollar when we were raising our 4 children years ago. We also knew that if we wanted to be good parents, it not only meant teaching them wrong from right, but how to live well and take care of their health for years to come.

Three things I use to tell my patients:

→ Health is a decision...
→ Working around a firm and committed decision can be done...
→ Excuses are plentiful when you want to be right...

Do you want to be "healthy and live the best life?"

- OR -

"Do you want to be right that things can't change and play Russian roulette with your health?"

What if you started to purchase healthier choices and just enough? I worked with several of my patients teaching them how to feed their families healthier meals on a budget.

Here is a true story of a remarkable and now healthier family...

I remember Dakota (name changed), a 54-year-old mother of 4 who was just diagnosed with Type II Diabetes, high blood pressure, high cholesterol and was 40+ pounds overweight. She now has Metabolic Syndrome. Her blood sugars had been borderline for about 2 years before she was diagnosed but she told me that she didn't even want to think about it before. Her mom died at

49 of kidney disease brought on by years of uncontrolled blood sugars.

Now she had to face the music...

Dakota came to me after being referred by her physician. She was angry with her new diagnosis' and came in thinking she was not going to be able to change her family's eating habits, let alone her own habits of eating poorly and consuming processed foods. Dakota was also convinced that there was no room in the budget to eat healthier.

So as we talked about her health, it was a tearful visit. She admitted that she was just scared and needed a lot of education and support. Dakota shared that she learned how to cook from her mom, who learned from her mom. After understanding that their cooking habits promoted disease instead of preventing it, she realized why her mom lived for years with uncontrolled blood sugars. Dakota had 4 children and 3 of her 4 children were overweight and the other child was obese, obviously she was now scared for them too.

These are the things we worked on:

- Dakota signed up and attended one of my healthy cooking classes.
- We worked on meal planning. Very important especially if on a budget. Meal planning prevents waste. Fast food and processed meals sometimes are a result of

not planning ahead and it becomes habitually convenient.

- Finding healthy recipes that worked for her family was a huge part of them eating healthy on a budget. Most recipes can be looked at and you can replace certain ingredients with healthier options. Dakota was pleased with several crock pot recipes that she found and this actually replaced many of her instant family meals. Not only was it easy, but they returned home after a long day to an incredibly tasty warm meal.
- Dakota learned how to take leftovers and create 1-2 additional meals which decreased the amount of time in the kitchen.
- She learned how to shop with a list. Make it a habit to ONLY shop for those items on your pre-planned menu and written list. You will spend so much less.
- Dakota cleaned her pantry out and organized it so all food items could be seen easily. She learned to go through her refrigerator and pantry before creating her shopping list so she didn't double buy. I taught her to grab the sale paper and see what items were on sale that they could build a healthy meal from. Seasonal fruits and veggies are cheaper and should be taken advantage of. Never overbuy anything (even if on sale) if it isn't a healthy food you eat often. Spending money on

weekly preplanned meals will keep you on budget.

- Dakota and her family lived about 14 miles from the grocery store. In the past, they went to the store once per week and without a list. The mistake was, they took everyone and went shopping before they ate dinner. So instead of one person perhaps making unhealthy choices, 6 people were throwing in processed foods and sweets right and left. And even with all that Dakota admitted that they frequented the gas station close to their home (very often) for last minute items. She agreed that made her food budget much higher because of the convenience cost.

- She learned that depending on how often you shop, if you should purchase fresh, frozen or canned. Only buy fresh if it can be eaten within a 3 to 5-day span (depending on the item possibly longer.) Otherwise, shoot for the frozen if possible. Canned goods have added sodium so depending on the items and recipes you are using whether frozen or canned should be purchased. Both equally as nutritious.

- Dakota learned to keep her spice shelf updated. Spices are great and can change the taste of the same item, like rice. One spice can create an Indian dish while another an Oriental dish. Also spices have a tremendous amount of nutrients in them.

My healthy pantry is full of spices that I use on a daily basis.

- Her family learned where their priorities were. They would look at healthy food as an expense they could not afford, yet they all spent money weekly in areas that was not health promoting. Things like manicures at a salon for 3 of them every other week. Instead, they bought a few polishes and supplies and had a "girl's night at home" every other week and painted each other's. They had cable which was great for family entertainment but also rented outside movies 4-6 times per month. Dakota started bringing her lunch to work 3 out of 5 days of the week. Her husband took his lunch 5 days a week and actually enjoyed it more. By the time we added up all the extra non-health promoting stuff they were spending $$ on, they had an additional $325 per month to spend on the foods they thought they could not afford. By working off a list and menu they had an additional $125 than they normally would spend on groceries. That was $500 they spent that they were not aware of. It's easy to do. They put $250 more towards healthier meals and $150 a month into a vacation account. They shared with me that they never had a real vacation. This savings was very motivating for them!

- I worked with Dakota for about nine months. Her children and husband joined her after she showed them that she was serious and making progress in her first month. Nutrition counseling was done for the whole family. You are rarely in it alone and as I told Dakota - "Fighting the fight alone is rough. Facing it together may put some strain on the family now, but illness is not easy to live with either". She hugged me and agreed.

- Nine months later, the whole family lost about 180+ pounds all together. Dakota was no longer on any medications and her family was active and moving in the right direction. When I asked her if eating healthy was more expensive, she smiles and says "if it's a priority you will make it happen". Dakota and her husband put effort into tweaking their entire family budget, cut out unnecessary spending, stopped shopping at the gas station, avoided fast food restaurants and put their health as a top priority!

Ask yourself, where do you have room in your food budget to create a healthier menu? You may have to do many of the things Dakota and her family did, but in the end it was worth it. A few dollars here and there add up. *Health cannot be ignored, it is and always will be our most precious commodity.* If you do ignore it, eventually you will not be able to ignore future diagnosis', medications and expensive medical tests.

"The doctor of the future will

no longer treat

the human frame with drugs,

but rather will cure

and prevent disease with nutrition."

~ Thomas Edison

Chapter 13

Heart Disease & Cholesterol

There is much in the news about cholesterol. Do this, don't do this, eat this, and don't eat that. Confused and not sure which direction to go? I totally understand. Confusion leads the average person to do NOTHING. Being a nurse who specialized in cardiac health for many years, I want to sum this up for you.

Get tested at least 1-2 times a year, depending on your medical history. If your health care provider, *based on lab test results*, tells you that your cholesterol is too high specifically for YOU. Don't make excuses, the results are there and make a decision to get those arteries healthy again regardless of how it happened.

Believe it. Admit it. Own it. Don't deny it. The biggest response most people give to their health care provider once they are told that their numbers are not good, is they try to "defend" themselves. Many times at my practice, I would hear "I eat so healthy", "I have no idea why it's that high", "My mom, dad, brother, cousin, etc., has cholesterol issues so I was bound to get it regardless of how I ate".   Again, don't make excuses and make a decision to get those arteries healthy again regardless of how it happened

Learn the basics about your good lipoprotein (HDL), the bad lipoprotein (LDL) and your triglycerides. Understanding the importance of cholesterol in our bodies is vital. Become a student of how your body processes lipids (fats). Don't become overwhelmed, just learn the basics. I would rather you put your energy in fixing it than reading every article on the web about cholesterol. Your doctor's office may be able to provide educational materials to explain the basics.

If your health care provider suggests you see a nutritionist or dietician, follow through. Even if it's for a couple of visits to ask questions and really understand how food, especially processed, high fat and high sugar foods affect your numbers. Or learn from reputable resources. Most people, believe it or not, have good intentions to follow a healthy diet but fall back into old habits. The support and great advice you would get from a specially trained dietary professional is priceless.

Learn the difference between foods, herbs and statins and how they decrease your cholesterol. Your health care practitioner may have you try diet and exercise first before placing you on a medication to lower your cholesterol. However, please understand that when a diabetic or someone with heart disease has questionable numbers, the best approach for that practitioner may be to use medications to decrease the inflammation as quickly as possible, lowering their patients potential risk. That would help his/her immediate inflammatory issues, getting it under control. Then those patients should follow a more natural approach (diet/exercise/herbs) if advised. Even though many people dislike using statins, besides lowering cholesterol, statins have a positive anti-inflammatory response that affects other organs in our bodies.

I am a BIG supporter of the diet/exercise/holistic approach, but it really does matter what co-morbidities you have. Spend time talking with your health care practitioner, you should really understand the reasons why they suggested you follow a certain treatment or dietary protocol. Cholesterol treatment is not a "one-size-fits-all."

Exercise. Walk. Move. Create a daily habit. Saying you opt for medication because you don't want to change the way you eat or want to exercise? That's stickin' thinkin'. You are fooling yourself. Exercise will positively affect your body in so many ways, not just improving cholesterol. If needed, get a personal trainer even for a few sessions, join a gym, or buy a treadmill. I am a huge supporter of powerwalking daily and using weights.

Remember, it's your health. The time to fix it is not when you are in the ICU with heart damage and hooked up to a monitor saying to yourself

"I could of...OR...I should of." We only have one life. Live well!

"Every single person in the world,

every culture, every language,

every country,

every person in the world

knows it;

you are what you eat.

FOOD does MATTER.

~ David Wolfe

Chapter 14

Seeds & Nuts for Longevity

Nuts and seeds contain healthy fats that are essential to your heart health and should be a part of your healthy aging diet. Consuming these little powerhouses can help you manage any internal inflammation. Seeds and nuts can help maintain the normal structure of every cell in your body. Choosing these types of healthy fats can lower cholesterol, decrease inflammation and perhaps add years to your life.

Many people eat nuts on a regular basis, however, seeds should not be ignored. They are packed with healthy fats, antioxidants, minerals, fiber and loaded with more protein than nuts. Including these little powerhouse seeds into your daily diet can be vital to healthy aging. Seeds also aid in the absorption of veggies, so throw some in with your stir fry for additional nutrition.

Nuts have cardiovascular benefits, aid in diabetes prevention and weight maintenance and are a quick treat for an afternoon snack. A single serving size is about a handful of nuts or about 1 ounce. Consuming a variety of nuts and seeds is imperative as they all contain different minerals, vitamins and ratios of healthy fats.

I purchase my nuts and seeds in their most natural state from health food stores and online. But if all you have is a Walmart in your town, purchase them there. Just try to get them without the added oils and salt. Nuts and seeds are high in caloric values, so take a handful out of the jar onto a small plate. It's very easy to over eat nuts at one setting. Even though they are healthy, you can over do a good thing. Your waistline will thank you.

Some of the most common SEEDS I eat and recommend are:

Flax seeds:

They are dark brown and are an excellent source of omega-3s. I eat ground flax seeds every day when I make my morning smoothie. Flax helps reduce the inflammation that can leads to migraine headaches and rheumatoid arthritis. The lignans in flaxseed promotes a healthy digestive system. One tablespoon has three grams of fiber. Because of the alpha-linolenic acid in flax it helps promote bone health therefore good to prevent osteoporosis. Flaxseed is a great heart health seed which may help lower blood pressure.

How do I use them? Overall, I recommend using flax every way you can. You can also make a flaxseed paste and use it in place of an egg when baking. I sprinkle my salads, stir-fry's, soups and avocado sandwiches with ground flax. If in doubt what to put it on, sprinkle it on just about anything.

Chia seeds:

Chia seeds are loaded with fiber which will aid in a healthy digestive system. This seed is powerful, one single serving has 18% of the recommended daily intake for calcium and also 27% of your daily need for phosphorus, which we know promotes bone health. It contains Omega-3 fatty acids which will help with long term heart health.

How do I use them? I take a quart jar, add about 4-5 tablespoons of Chia seeds and add filtered water. Put a lid on and shake it well. Then about every 5 minutes I re-shake it. It will form a smooth thick liquid (in about 10-15 minutes). I place it into the fridge and use it in my morning smoothie. A whole jar will last you over a dozen smoothies. Add as little or as much as you like. A tablespoon or two is my norm. I also make delicious chia puddings which are super healthy for the whole family. I sprinkle the whole seeds into a variety of salads, veggie lasagna and soups. There are so many great things you can do to include the Chia seed into your diet.

Hemp seeds:

What I love about hemp hearts (shelled seeds) is that they are a complete protein. They're loaded with protein, healthy fats (mainly omega-3s), vitamin E, and minerals like magnesium and zinc. Hemp promotes a healthy complexion because it contains both Vitamin A and E. Hemp helps internal organs work better, like your nervous system, it helps your body metabolize fats and promotes brain function. It is full of soluble, insoluble fiber and essential fatty acids. This seed is deliciously nutty, slightly sweet with a pleasant crunchy texture that you can add to so many different things.

What do I do with them? I add hemp into my morning smoothie as a great way to start my day. I make homemade protein bars, muffins and use them over salads to increase the nutrient content of the salad, in soups and sprinkle over homemade frozen banana non-dairy ice cream. Love my hemp...

Sesame seeds:

My favorite snack seeds. They are full of essential minerals such as zinc, iron, manganese, copper, phosphorus and calcium which promotes bone health. Sesame seeds promote a healthy immune system because of its antioxidant capacity it fights free radicals in our body which can cause cancer. These seeds also contain iron which is necessary for good blood health.

What do I do with them? I use sesame seeds in many ways especially cooked dishes because they add texture to baked goods. I roll black sesame seeds (they contain 60% more calcium than hulled white sesame seeds) into my vegetarian sushi rolls for color, taste and superb health. I throw a handful into my stir-fries and salads and like to make homemade hummus with ground sesame seeds. Lots to do with this tasty seed.

Pumpkin seeds:

Pumpkin seeds (pepitas) are full of so many great nutrients that making them a frequent snack would be a superb health choice. They contain protein, B vitamins, vitamin K, vitamin E, phosphorus, magnesium, copper, manganese, zinc and iron. Pepitas can help you sleep better because of the L-tryptophan they contain and they also reduce inflammation and protect you from osteoporosis. This small green seed does all this and more.

What do I do with them? I create a great granola with many types of seeds, pepitas being one of the main ingredients. I enjoy baking them when they are fresh right out of the pumpkin, you can create many tasty flavors depending on the spice you use. Especially around the holidays, I like to make dozens of organic breads (banana, pumpkin, sweet potato, etc.) and share them with others. When I bake organic pumpkin bread I place the seeds on the top for a nice healthy look and they taste great. I make a sweet butternut squash soup and sprinkle pepitas on the top. I add them to soups and stews. If you have not tasted or used pepitas before, try a small amount and experiment. You can buy them already shelled at your health food store and in local groceries. I believe you will love them.

Sunflower seeds:

They have been used by Native Americans for more than 5,000 years. They used the seeds as a food and an oil source, but also used the flowers, roots and stems. These amazing seeds are used for detox and to cleanse the body. Like other seeds, they contain so many nutrients and needed vitamins in fact just ¼ cup provides you with almost all the Vitamin E you need in a day. Sunflower seeds are a powerhouse when helping our cells inhibit cancer cells. Because of the selenium in sunflower seeds, they help our DNA repair system. Just knowing that it helps with inflammation and cell health is a reason to incorporate this seed into your diet a couple times per week. Magnesium is rich in this seed, which results in lowering your blood pressure and decreasing muscle tension, migraines and fatigue.

How do I use them? I enjoy a handful of mild nutty sunflower seeds to take care of my afternoon hunger. Of course, I create a granola with them. I sprinkle some into my hot oatmeal for extra taste and nutrition. You can also add sunflower seeds to your favorite salad recipe. Bottom line, seeds bring us great health, use them as much as possible. A little sprinkle here and sprinkle there and you've continued to decrease the inflammation in that healthy body of yours!

A little about NUTS and some of the most common nuts I eat and recommend. Nuts are such an underrated snack. My favorites (everyone has their own) are almonds, walnuts, cashews, and pistachios. But there are so MANY more to enjoy. Nuts can help lower cholesterol, improve your heart health and studies have shown they may even lower your cancer risk. Some people totally avoid nuts because they are a high calorie nutritious snack. As a health nut (no pun intended), I incorporate nuts into my daily diet, I just know when to stop. Remember, just because something is labeled healthy doesn't mean it is low calorie.

Great story to share...

Karan (name changed), a patient of mine gained about 20 lbs. over a 3-month period and came to see me because she no longer fit into her work clothes and could not afford new ones. During the interview process, I asked her many questions. Her father had a heart attack at age 60. It threw her for a loop and she wanted to do better with her meals and snacks. She admitted she knew so little about nutrition or reading labels and her mom cooked only from mixes and processed boxes (like hamburger helper, etc.)

Karan was a frequent "drive thru" addict and knew that those types of foods may add to her potential heart disease. She hated fast food salads and if she went to restaurant she hated eating alone, so in her mind she made a plan to just "snack" healthy items all day. Karan found at the grocery store a nut/dried fruit snack that said "Great for Cardiac Health" on its label.

She recently had changed jobs and now drives at least 15 hours per week to get from location to location. She initially thought that the long distance sitting was adding to her weight gain but could not change that, so she would walk an extra 30 minutes a day to offset it, which was a fairly good plan for that part.

On the next visit I had Karan bring in her cans and bags of nuts/dried fruits and healthy snacks. I also had her keep a very accurate food journal. What I found was a "marketing manufacturers dream." If it said healthy, Karan bought it! Out of all the snacks she bought, the nuts/dried fruit mixture was her favorite. The can had a symbol of a heart on it and they boasted the nutrition on the front. However, Karan was consuming about 500-800 extra calories of nuts/dried fruit per day adding to her caloric intake, which was definitely more than she should have for her height and weight.

You may judge Karan and say "didn't she read the nutrition label and eat only the serving size it recommends?" Interestingly, I have found over the past decade that most of my patients would admit that they look at the labels but have no idea how it to make it work for them. US labels are based on a person who consumes about 2000 calories per day. It's not individualized so people become confused. In my cooking classes, I teach how to read AND interpret a food label to make it work for YOU. Many attendees from the class admitted they knew very little to help themselves.

Karan registered for one of my healthy cooking classes about a week later and her life changed. How something simple as cooking a healthy meal can be overwhelming for someone who has never been taught the right way. I learned a long time ago not to judge, just teach with passion and encourage.

We came up with easy and healthy snacks to travel with which included nuts/dried fruit but in small amounts. Karan not only lost the 20 lbs. she gained, but lost an additional 20 that had been hanging around since her son's birth 3 years prior. I was proud of her because so many people know what to do, but even when taught, do not follow through. Karan is a success story.

Sooooo... Don't let Karan's story scare you. Nuts are such a wonderful superfood. Avoiding them because of a higher calorie is unnecessary. I add nuts to my smoothie every morning so I am assured to benefit from all they have to offer. Then once a day I may eat a small amount with some seeds and fresh fruit for a snack.

Walnuts:

Wow, the best of the best when it comes to nutrition. Walnuts are the richest in omega-3 fatty acids. This high prestigious job the walnut has helps "fight inflammation" and therefore protects your body from cellular damage that can cause premature aging, heart disease and cancer. I learned a long time ago at a nutrition seminar I attended that the walnut possesses very powerful omega-3 fatty acids that are good for our brains. Look at the shape of the walnut...it is almost identical to the shape of our brain. No one there will ever forget that one!

What do I do with them? I include walnuts into my power smoothie in the morning in small amounts. I throw a few onto a salad with some dried cranberries (a great mix). I love to use them in bran muffin recipes. I stuff acorn squash with brown rice, apples, spices, cranberries and walnuts. Delicious. I bake pears with walnuts and raisins. I throw them in wraps and use my imagination as I cook. I always ask myself, how can I make a dish healthier, even by a nut or two?

Almonds:

This eye shaped nut contains the most fiber than other nuts and is rich in a powerful antioxidant, Vitamin E. Excellent nut for your digestive system. Almonds can be a part of helping you to lose weight or stabilize your blood sugar. It obviously is heart healthy and can help to decrease your bad cholesterol (LDL). Nuts, including almonds help your immune system and as we age this is a vital part of eating well. I used almonds as part of my patients "Plate Plan" I developed at my practice. Not only did individuals lose weight because of the combination of healthy foods that I suggested they eat, but 8-10 almonds kept their hunger at bay.

What do I do with them? I shred them with other ingredients, then use them to top things like I would cheese. Like on sandwiches, soups and salads. Experiment, it's fun. I take -> a cup raw almonds, 2 Tbls of nutritional yeast (I use Braggs), add 1 tsp garlic powder and ½ tsp of mineral salt. I put it into my Nutri Bullet (you can use a food processor or blender) and blend it until you get a consistency you like. Wanting to create a different type of dish, I used the above recipe and put it on a cooked potato along with dried tomatoes. It really does add flavor and you avoid the saturated animal fat from cheese.

Obviously a few almonds taste great on top of any kind of salad. Four to five almonds go into my smoothie every morning. I create a nut crust for baking and also put them in my oatmeal along with organic cinnamon and a fresh apple or banana. When making buckwheat pancakes, add some crushed or shredded almonds to the mix. Almonds can make fantastic healthy cookies and muffins. There really is unlimited ways to get your Vitamin E.

Cashews:

This kidney shaped nut can help improve your memory and protect you against age-related memory loss because of the all magnesium they have in them. They give you a brain power boost.

Cashews are incredibly high in zinc and iron which helps your immune system and vision. They help our bones and nerves. Cashews have a lower fat content than most other nuts and contain monounsaturated fats which are heart-healthy. So as we age, keeping a few cashews around can be a good...no GREAT thing. I do not use this nut in my smoothie as I like to relish its delicious flavor alone, perhaps for a snack eating the whole nut or in a cashew butter.

What do I do with them? I enjoy all nut butters, cashew included. I put some on celery or fresh apples. Combining cashews with other nuts and dried fruits makes a super healthy snack. If you add cashews to vegetable stir fry's (which I love), throw them in at the end, just before removing the pan from the stove. Cashew butter can also be used to cook in many hot dishes to create a wonderful sauce. Keep a can of cashews in your spice cabinet, and get creative!

Pistachios:

Pistachios are one of the oldest nuts and most commonly used, going back to 6000 BC. They contain vitamins, minerals, fats and protein. The health benefits of pistachios are almost endless because they are so high in a variety of different nutrients. They are one of the few nuts that contain almost all of the nutrients required by humans for a healthy and complete longevity. Pistachios have a multitude of health benefits, such as; protection against diabetes, they are great for heart health, improves digestion and blood pressure issues. Many people love pistachios for the weight management it seems to help with. A pistachio tree can take up to 10 years to produce their first crop.

My personal experience with this old nut...lol. We moved into a new home last year, the back yard was large, lots of room to breathe, to write and to meditate in. It had a plum tree, sage bushes and two patios to enjoy while looking up at the beautiful Sacramento Mountains that are literally steps away. We live in the desert so being blessed with all of this was actually priceless.

In our front yard, we were blessed to have three VERY large pistachios trees, one male and two females. We learned how to care of them, when to pick, when to prune, I had no idea before all this. It was fun to learn and I felt like an organic farmer! Interestingly, the male grows "beautiful blooms" on his branches in the spring, then just stays green throughout the summer. The female grows the actual "nuts." Mother nature definitely has nutty humor! Pistachios are harvested in the fall. We were incredibly blessed to have both female trees FULL of nuts, over 150 lbs. to harvest. We learned how to shake the nuts off the trees and how to prune them in the winter so when they return they are full of more delicious nuts.

Fruit and nut bearing trees are a blessing to have within arm's reach especially for a health nut like myself. Next door, our neighbors Teresa and Jack have apricot and pomegranate trees. Over the past year we have kindly shared our fresh fruit and nuts with each other. Life is good.

What do I do with them? First, my husband made some incredible Pistachio Brittle in many different flavors. He's never made any type of brittle before but the batches turned out like an expert bake them. We have shared brittle with many of our friends and family over the holidays. I love to bake pistachio bread. It's so easy to add them to desserts. You can also add them to any healthy cookie recipe or create a pistachio crust then fill with your favorite pie. I made a Pumpkin Pie using ground pistachios for the crust along with a delicious Pear and Pistachio Crisp. You can buy pistachios just about everywhere, in the shell or shelled.

There are many other kinds of nuts and over the past several years I found that everyone has their favorite kind. No matter what kind you love, find ways to include them in your daily meals in small amounts. Here a few and there a few will add huge health benefits to add to your EFOY basket!

"Health is not valued till

sickness comes."

~ Dr. Thomas Fuller

Chapter 15

Oils & Cooking

Cooking oils have been around for thousands of years. In the past 100 years it has changed because of the processing and chemicals used. One thing I do want to stress is that oil is a fat, and fat calories are still fat calories regardless of the type of oil you use. So, you should use the least amount of fat possible to prepare your foods while still getting the greatest amount of taste and health benefits. People use oils for a variety of dishes, some hot and some cold.

I personally use as little oil as I can. When I do it's usually an avocado or coconut oil. There are days or even weeks that go by without me using any at all. I use substitutes such as flaxseed and applesauce to cook with if oil is needed in baked goods. Remember, unsaturated fats are best. They can help round out a diet rich in fruits, vegetables, legumes, nuts, seeds and whole grains. Limiting animal and saturated fats and totally avoiding trans-fats whenever possible should be your healthy longevity goal.

Because the media has talked so much about "healthy olive oils", etc., many American will actually add it to their diets routinely thinking that they are improving their health. I do NOT recommend this. If you are going to use any oil, use it sparingly or *just what the recipe calls for*. Each oil has its own taste, and texture, so picking the right one is important for the end result of the dish you are preparing.

Here is a list of the types of oils there are and what it's best used in. When I do use oil, I make sure that it is organic and I never cook any hotter than their "smoke points" (see below).

Avocado – frying, sautéing, marinades

Canola – baking, sautéing, light cooking, sauces

Coconut – baking, sautéing, light dishes

Flax – dips, marinades, dressings

Grapeseed – sautéing, salads, salsa, dips, drizzled

Olive – sautéing, dips, marinades, drizzled

Palm – baking, frying

Peanut – frying, dips, marinades, stir fries

Sesame – frying, sautéing, dips, marinades, stir fries, sauces

Sunflower – baking, sautéing

Walnut – dressing, dips, marinades

Wheat Germ – dressing, dips, marinades

The SMOKE POINT. What does the smoke point of a cooking oil mean? The smoke point is the temperature that causes oil to start smoking.

When it reaches a certain temperature it can produce toxic fumes and harmful free radicals (cancer causing). If an oil overheats, I would suggest throwing it out along with the food you overheated. Take special care of which oil that you are using. Usually, every label has their smoke point on it. Always use the lowest amount of heat to attain the best results! A good rule of thumb is that the more refined the oil, the higher the smoke point.

"If you change the way you

look at things,

the things you look at change."

~ Dr. Wayne Dyer

Chapter 16

Good Fats -vs- Bad Fats
Help I'm Confused!

You've heard a lot about fats lately. Don't let all the articles confuse you. I am going to make it very simple for you. There are 3 major players in our dietary health: Carbohydrates, Protein and Fats. Fats add to the flavor of our dishes including texture.

Here are the four different types of fats:

Monounsaturated: are the healthiest and known for being heart healthy. Some examples are avocado, nuts, olives, sesame seeds and nuts (almonds, cashews, hazelnuts, macadamia nuts, peanuts, pecans) and a natural peanut butter (check the ingredients and only purchase the one that says just peanuts and salt). I actually prefer nut butters other than peanut. Almond butter being my favorite. Try different ones, you may be surprised how good many of them are.

Polyunsaturated: become rancid easier especially when exposed to sunlight. Never keep past expiration date. This includes walnuts, seeds such as sunflower, sesame seeds, pumpkin seeds and flaxseed. Fatty fish such as sardines, salmon, tuna, herring and trout. Non-GMO soymilk and tofu are also great sources. Cooking at high heat with some monounsaturated or polyunsaturated oils can damage the fat. Not healthy, nor safe.

Saturated: have long shelf and you can cook at higher temperatures. Found in animal dishes. For many years, we've been told that the simplest way to prevent heart disease is to replace saturated fats for their healthier, unsaturated counterparts. Wrong. The newest dietary information we have suggests that things are not just that simple.

Some dieticians and nutritionists feel that manufactured vegetable oils should not be included as "good" fats. When being processed, it can damage the oil and when that happens it can transform the fatty acids into a dangerous trans-fat.

I cannot stress enough how important the smoking point is or storing oils inappropriately. Good fats can become bad if heat, light, or oxygen damages it. Polyunsaturated fats must be refrigerated and kept in a container where the light does not affect it. Throw out oils, seeds, or nuts after they begin to smell or taste bitter as they are spoiled and can do more harm than good.

Trans fat: Experts will say that this fat is the very worst kind. Trans fats are chemically altered fats which are found in partially hydrogenated oils. Hydrogen is injected under high heat and high pressure. They invented this type of fat decades ago to help extend shelf life. As our food industry grew, they were looking for ways to extend the shelf life of processed foods in the grocery stores and at home.

Did you ever wonder why or how many "snack foods" you eat can last on your shelves for years? When you open up the package, it smelled, looked and taste like it was made yesterday? Answer, by using a trans-fat. Some examples are: Baked goods, fried foods, crackers, chips, cookies, breakfast cereals, margarine, cookies, etc. If it says in the list of ingredients that it has a "partially hydrogenated" anything in it – STAY AWAY!

One of the many health issues I have with my patients consuming this type of fat is that it lowers their good cholesterol (HDL) and raises their bad cholesterol (LDL). Consuming trans fats have proven to increase the risk of coronary artery disease. Mix that with an inflammatory diet and you have a heart attack waiting to happen. In 2006, it had to be listed on the food label. Problem is, not every food item is affected by the law so it's up to the consumer to ask or research it. Pain in the ---- I know, but you are protecting your health along with your family's health.

The FDA has been more involved in promoting companies to decrease the use of these chemically process fats. It will take a year or two or three for compliance but at least we are on the right path. Some health food stores will not sell products with trans fats, so it's up to you to ask, research and read the labels in the meantime.

Most people already know about the benefits of omega-3 fatty acids that I just wrote about, particularly EPA/DHA from fish and other sources. However, the typical American diet (SAD) contains way too much omega-6 fatty acids. Our goals are to reduce this type of fat in our diet. Sources of omega-6s include most vegetable oils such as soybean oil, corn oil, safflower oil, along with eggs and poultry.

There is one omega-6, however, called gamma linolenic acid (GLA) that has been shown to fight disease. New research has shown what it does to combat a multitude of inflammatory diseases. Balancing a larger amount of Omega 3 -vs- a smaller amount of Omega 6 can be a challenge for many because Omega 6 runs rampantly through snacks and items that people love to eat. This type of fat can become addictive to your taste buds. Studies have shown that omega-6 fatty acids should be consumed in a 1:1 ratio to omega-3, even though the diet of many individuals today is at a ratio of about 16:1. Scary for their short and long term health.

Anything with "partially hydrogenated" oil listed as an ingredient should be a red flag and avoid consuming it. Feeding these type of food to your children just sets them up for health issues early in life. MANY commercially baked goods and packaged items contain trans fats. It may not say it on the first half of the label, but if you see "partially hydrogenated" ANYWHERE on the label, put it immediately back on the shelf.

Bottom line...

1.	Read all food labels.

2.	Eliminate fried foods.

3.	Limit the use of oils and when you do use them, pay attention to the smoke point and storage of it.

4.	Eat Omega-3 foods every day.

5.	Cook real food, convenience is great but your health is at stake. There are great recipes in my new cookbook *"Eat The Way YOU Want to Look"* that will show you how quickly you can put together a delicious plant based dish.

"What is called genius is the abundance

of life and health."

~ Henry David Thoreau

Chapter 17

Healthy Longevity...

Omega-3 Fatty Acids...

Super Fats for YOUR Brain!

Our brains thrive on fats. Omega-3 fatty acids play a very important role in cognitive function. Our ability to remember and solves problems along with emotional health is tied to great nutrition. Protecting ourselves against one of the major aging concerns – dementia and Alzheimer's. Omega-3's can also help decrease the inflammation from joint disease and the rest of our bodies. It also helps balance our moods and fatigue that can happen as we age.

According to the GazetteNet.com, "With over five million Americans currently living with Alzheimer's disease, researchers are examining which dietary fats may help prevent dementia. Olivia Okereke at Brigham & Women's Hospital tested how different types of fats affect cognition and memory in women. Over the course of four years, she found that women who consumed high amounts of monounsaturated fats had better overall cognitive function and memory."

"A study by researchers from Laval University in Quebec revealed similar findings: Diets high in monounsaturated fats increased the production and release of the neurotransmitter acetylcholine, which is critical for learning and memory. The loss of acetylcholine production in the brain has been associated with Alzheimer's disease."

"Unfortunately, canola oil, which is high in monounsaturated fats in its natural form, is often hydrogenated so it can stay fresh longer in processed foods. Partially hydrogenated oils—also known as Trans fats—were shown to be detrimental to memory in a recent University of California San Diego study. "Trans fats increase the shelf life of the food but reduce the shelf life of the person," reports study author Beatrice Golomb."

Did you just read what I read? Reduce "MY shelf life?" – NO WAY! Of course, a well-rounded balanced diet with plenty of fruits and vegetables may still be the best way to stay healthy. But it's good to know that good fats won't harm you. In fact, it might help you live a healthier, more productive life.

I suggest these 9 healthy fats to use in your diet:

> ➔ Avocados
> ➔ Dark Chocolate
> ➔ Fatty Fish (if not vegetarian or vegan)
> ➔ Nuts
> ➔ Chia, Pumpkin and Hemp Seeds
> ➔ Coconuts and Coconut Oil
> ➔ Flaxseed

→ Dark Greens such as Kale, Spinach and Brussels Sprouts.

→ Beans have Omega-3

As you can see by drinking my "Edible Fountain of Youth Smoothie" every morning, you will get the majority of your Omega-3's out of the way for the day. Your brain, heart and immune system will thank you!!!

"You are what you eat, so don't be

Fast... Easy...

Cheap... or

Fake!

~ Unknown Author

Chapter 18

Super Healthy Grains

Grains, a great health food, is an essential part of maintaining a healthy lifestyle. It is an easy way to create a diet that is healthier, richer and more balanced. Grains are easy to cook and can enhance a dishes flavor and nutrient load especially when mixed with other superfoods such as vegetables and spices.

I realize that some people cannot eat whole wheat and gluten containing foods and if it truly is a health reason, then I understand. There are many grains left to consume. I have found over the years that most people do not eat grains because they really do not know what to do with them or how to cook with them. The internet these days is a great resource along with recipes in my new cookbook, "Eat The Way YOU Want to Look."

There are three ways grains end up...

Whole, refined and enriched.

When a grain is considered **whole** it hasn't had any of their edible parts (bran, germ, and endosperm) removed by milling. Milling removes many of the essential nutrients.

Whole grains contain complex carbohydrates, proteins, antioxidants, dietary fiber, B vitamins, folic acid and trace minerals. Whole grains are better sources of fiber and other important nutrients, such as selenium, potassium and magnesium. They are also low in fat and can help reduce the risk of: heart disease, bad cholesterol levels, obesity, metabolic syndrome, type 2 diabetes and some cancers. Whole grain diets have also been proven to improve bowel health by promoting healthy bacteria to grow in the colon therefore producing healthier BM's. A healthy colon will impact your immune system in a positive way.

Refined grains are milled whole grains that had their bran and germ removed by milling to improve shelf life. Examples of refined grains include white flour, white rice and white bread. Many processed foods such as breads, crackers, cereals, and desserts are made with refined grains, too.

Enriched means that some of the nutrients were lost during processing then placed back into the product. Some enriched grains have lost their B vitamins so they literally add them back.

Fortifying means that the manufacturer added additional nutrients that don't occur naturally in that particular food. Most refined grains are also enriched, and many enriched grains are fortified with other vitamins and minerals. It's very common to see folic acid and iron added. Whole grains may or may not be fortified. By reading the label you will know what you are purchasing and consuming.

Examples of some whole grains are:

Quinoa

Wild Rice

Whole Rye

Brown rice, Black Rice, Red Rice

100% Whole Wheat Flour

Bulgur Wheat

Whole Oats

Farro

Millet

Barley

Buckwheat

Kamut

Spelt

And several others. Best way to try a new whole grain is to search the internet on a few healthy cooking sites, find a "new grain recipe" you have never tried and make it. You can usually purchase the majority of every day grains in the grocery store. If not, try your local health food store - who usually has big bins full of grains.

Or order thru Amazon, they have just about anything you would need!

Several years ago, I added one new grain a month until I found my absolute favorites. Cooking grains are not difficult and can be made ahead and stored in the fridge in sealed containers for several days, then tossed into salads, stir-fry's, soups and much more.

My favorite grains that I cook with often are: Wild rice (actually a grass), black rice, brown rice, quinoa, whole oats and farro. One of my favorite kitchen appliances is a rice cooker – oh my gosh, so many different grains you can cook in there and NOT burn. Every grain needs to be cooked and you can find those directions on the bag it comes in or if needed google it online. Also if using a rice cooker, refer to the cooker's instructions to see what it can cook and for how long.

Live Bread: I like to eat an Organic Sprouted Bread (i.e. Ezekiel Brand) because:

- It is a complete protein source, contains 18 amino acids (9 of them essential amino acids).
- The bread easily digests.
- It absorbs minerals much better. Minerals such as iron, calcium, magnesium, copper and zinc.
- Sprouted bread has an increased amount of vitamin C along with B2, 5 and 6.

- Good amount of fiber with a great taste.

If you have never tried sprouted bread, it's worth getting a loaf. You can purchase it in just about any health food store and some big chain supermarkets do carry it. You must keep it refrigerated and *many sell it in the freezer section.* I take out a couple slices as needed.

One of my favorite open sandwiches is toasting a slice of bread lightly, adding a few slices of fresh avocado along with a tomato, throw a little black pepper on it and you have yourself a super healthy snack.

"The food you eat can either be the safest

and most powerful form of medicine

OR

the slowest form of poison."

~ Ann Wigmore

Chapter 19

Processed Foods,
Accelerating the Aging Process
and Animal Protein

Recently, the World Health Organization has announced that processed meats are as detrimental to our health as other carcinogens. As I spread my knowledge for good nutrition, I try to focus on plant based meals without being pushy towards meat eaters because I realize that what we eat is a choice. However, with this announcement, I HIGHLY advise that all processed meats (i.e. hotdogs, pepperoni, sandwich meats, sausage, bacon, etc.) be avoided or minimized in adult diets and TOTALLY avoided in children's diets especially as toddlers and children. Too much is at risk. Parents want to do the best for their children, not consuming the kinds of processed meats listed above is part of being a great parent.

Studies have shown where mothers and infants are tested at birth and both have several chemicals within their systems. This is interesting because being pregnant you try to eat well and take care of yourself for the baby you are carrying. So if some of our children come into this world with blood levels already affected, why add more to them?

Foods really affects our little ones whether we feed them nutritious meals or instant-prepared meals with very little nutrition. What we feed them today, while they are growing definitely affects their brains and bodies, now and in the future. There are so many studies about childhood illnesses being brought on by their exposure to chemicals in the air, through their delicate skin and the meals they are provided.

My thoughts are – we avoid many things we think may cause our children harm. We protect them in so many ways as loving parents. Unfortunately, we "trust" our food industry and our government to keep us safe. We also trust that the food industry is passing safe laws and monitoring carcinogens. I would love to believe that to be true. Unfortunately, there is a lot of politics in our food industry. Look at other countries, they prohibit many of the foods that our FDA thinks is safe and is currently being sold in our country.

Below is part of an internet article that may open your eyes from *"Eat This, Not That!"*

"It's no secret that our food system is broken. Any country that allows us to unknowingly eat wood chips, yoga mats, human hair, beetle shells, beaver sex glands, and all number of synthetic chemicals isn't looking out for our nutritional interests."

"And while the USA is busy labeling pizza a vegetable, other countries are taking steps to protect their people from dangerous food-like products. Here are some foods that you can find in your grocery store that are banned in other countries."

In the article, it discusses carcinogenic additives in many of the foods you may be consuming. They also cover how food dyes are banned in many other countries but used frequently in America. Food dyes may have an adverse effect on the activity and attention in children. Milk with growth hormones are banned but again used here. And the chicken we think is so safe can be exposed to chlorinated water baths, rinses, and mists as an antimicrobial treatment.

If you'd like to read a copy of the article above, here is the link:

http://www.eatthis.com/american-foods-products-banned-in-other-countries

FYI...

The EU (European Union) countries consist of Austria, Belgium, Bulgaria, Croatia, Republic of Cyprus, Czech Republic, Denmark, Estonia, Finland, France, Germany, Greece, Hungary, Ireland, Italy, Latvia, Lithuania, Luxembourg, Malta, Netherlands, Poland, Portugal, Romania, Slovakia, Slovenia, Spain, Sweden and the UK.

If all of the health experts in these countries have banned these products, what is our health system (the Food and Drug Administration) thinking? Or not thinking. Are we driven by those who write the rules and are influenced by large manufacturers? Interesting. Humans are all alike. EU consist of 28 different countries, along with several health specialists in each one. I tend to go with the masses who are trying to protect their citizens.

Bottom line; food dyes, additives and the way processed foods are prepared in our country is affecting our nation's health. Be a part of making a difference and protect the ones you love.

What foods can age you faster?

- Sugar, sugary foods and certain starchy foods may cause blood sugar spikes over time, and that can increase those age-accelerating compounds called AGEs.

  Instead of sugar, consider using a natural sweetener like Stevia. This can dramatically help you control your blood sugar response and thereby help slow the aging process.

  See Chapter 25 on Dark Chocolate. It can be a tasty part of healthy aging and it's how I satisfy my sweet tooth. There is about 2 grams of sugar in every 1-2 small squares of dark chocolate. FYI: Your typical cake or ice cream can have 30-80 grams of age-accelerating sugar.

- White rice, white bread and white potatoes can have significant impact on your blood sugar thereby increasing the formation of AGEs (they speed up the aging process) in your body. If you are going to eat these foods, eat them in small portions balancing them with healthy fats and protein to slow your blood sugar response down.

- High fructose corn syrup (HFCS), corn oil, corn chips and corn cereals. Some people eat these foods daily and are most at risk. It has become one of the worst food additives in America. Starchy foods such as cereals containing corn can impact your blood sugar and drive up the AGEs in your body accelerating the aging process. Mix that with affecting your heart and brain health and it's something to consider seriously avoiding. So many people consume foods that have HFCS without realizing it and you may be one of them. Read the label of everything you put into your internal engine. These foods also contribute excessive amounts of omega-6 fatty acids to your diet, which leads to inflammation and oxidation within your body.

- Vegetable oils. Too many people use oils like water in the foods that they prepare. Because vegetable oils are so processed, they can contain chemicals and increase oxidation which is NOT what we want in our internal engines. This processing can be very inflammatory, producing free radicals and causing serious health issues. It can contribute to the aging process even faster which is what we are trying to slow down.

In Chapter 15, "Oils & Cooking", I discuss the wide variety and what they are used in but also talk about using the minimum amounts. The oils I do use when needed are healthy oils and fats such as organic avocado oil, organic virgin coconut oil and occasionally organic olive oil.

I really feel like in today's world the media, the oil manufacturers and their marketing departments have given us the idea that you should add oils and lots of them to your daily diet. Unfortunately, even though there are some oils that can offer definite health benefits, *does not mean to over use or to add to a dish when you normally would not.*

"Health is like money; we never

have a true idea

of its value until we lose it."

~ Josh Billings

Chapter 20

Dietary Protein
Is Much MORE
Than Just Animal Meat

As a vegetarian for many years, (vegan now) I get asked pretty often what I eat for my protein. If you study nutrition, you would find out that all food sources have protein, some more than others, but all do. Animal protein is tied to many health issues. Even though this book is not going to cover this specifically, I suggest if healthy longevity is what you are after, then omitting any red meat is highly suggested.

I am not asking you to become vegan, we all make our own choices. I am recommending that you consider creating a lifestyle where your diet is mainly plant based and perhaps the animal meat your "side dish." If you want the real answer to longevity, then working towards this way of eating will not only help your brain, heart and skin but will help you to avoid major disease as you age.

Protein is the building blocks of life. In our body, it breaks down into amino acids which in turn promotes cell growth and repair. You know that animal products such as dairy, meat and eggs are one source of protein. Sadly, this type of protein can also be high in saturated fat and heart clogging cholesterol. What many people do not realize is that you absolutely do not need to eat animal protein (meat, cheese, eggs, milk) to get your protein needs met.

Women need approximately 35-45 grams of protein per day. Men need between 45-60, *all depending on their size and of course their level of daily activity.* For healthy longevity, I suggest you get as many plant based proteins into your diet daily.

These are some great vegetarian and vegan protein sources, along with some tips on how to include them into your diet.

- Beans – many different types of beans. Black, kidney, white, pinto, etc. All of them have their own special taste and texture but all have high amounts of protein. As an example, 2 cups of kidney beans, contain approximately 26 grams. Great part, you don't have to cook beans from scratch to reap their nutritional benefits. Purchasing them in bulk and soak them overnight to cook in the morning is great. However, for convenience, purchasing them canned is easier, quicker and just as tasty. I suggest you check to be sure that the cans are not lined with BPA. I use beans in hundreds of recipes because of their flavor and versatile texture. You can throw them into soups, stir fry's, make bean burgers, decorate salads and use them endlessly in many recipes.

- Chia Seeds - has 4.7 grams per ounce in 2 tablespoons. Chia seeds are an incredibly easy way to add protein and fiber to almost ANY recipe. I sprinkle Chia seeds over my salads, you can stir them into your yogurt or oatmeal, or my favorite thing to do is blend a couple tablespoons of Chia paste into my "Edible Fountain of Youth" smoothie every morning. Because they plump up and take on a gelatinous texture when soaked in a liquid, you can create yummy creamy puddings out of this versatile seed.

- Chickpeas – this power house legume is also known as a garbanzo beans. They contain 7.3 grams of protein per half cup. They are also high in fiber and low in calories. Chickpeas can be tossed into soups, salads, toasted in the oven or pureed into a delicious hummus. I frequently take a whole-wheat flatbread, spread on some homemade hummus (or you can purchase it at your local grocery store already prepared), add some veggies and you have a great lunch sandwich. I love it with a bowl of warm soup to create a healthy little meal.

- Edamame – a versatile and delicious soybean still in the pod. It contains 8.4 grams of protein per half cup that can be served hot or cold and many people sprinkle the pods with salt for a snack. They are great as an appetizer, snack or remove the shells and add it to a stir fry for taste and a colorful green addition. For convenience, you can purchase a bag of just the soybeans out of their pods. I always keep an extra bag in the freezer!

- Greens – leafy greens don't have as much protein as legumes and nuts, however, many do contain significant amounts of protein along with antioxidants and importantly a heart healthy fiber. Amino acids can come from consuming a wide variety of different types of vegetables. For an example, just 2 cups of raw spinach contain 2.1 grams of protein and one cup of chopped broccoli contains 8.1 grams. Greens really rock and should be part of your daily diet at every meal. Fix them as salads, throw them into soups, and stir fry's, sandwiches and wraps.
- Green peas – have 7.9 grams per cup. They are actually in the legume family and has about the same amount of protein as milk. It is great to throw into salads or warm up as a side dish.
- Hemp - has approximately 10 grams in 3 tbls. You can find this protein in some cereals and trail mixes, or you can buy hemp seeds and add them to smoothies, warm cereals such as oatmeal, or baked goods. Hemp milk is even lower in calories than skim milk and can be a dairy-free way

to add protein to your diet. I add some to my "Edible Fountain of Youth" smoothie every morning!

- Quinoa – has 8.1 grams per cup. Quinoa is a seed that actually contains all 9 essential amino acids that our bodies need for growth and repair. You can add Quinoa to just about anything. I add it to my homemade soups, vegetarian chili, stir fry's or throw into a salad.

- Non Dairy Milks – Nut and soy milks can be great additions to any diet. If you are lactose intolerant you may have already tried some of the different types. It has become a real trend to use nondairy milks by millions of people and considering some of the negative issues cow's milk has, this is a great choice. Read the labels (like everything else) and watch out for the added sugars, added carrageenan (totally AVOID) and flavors. Soy milk has the most protein, at 5 to 8 grams per 8 ounces. Almond, hemp, and rice milk contain approximately 1 gram per cup.

- Nut Butters - Nuts contain healthy fats and protein, making them a valuable part of a plant-based diet. Almonds, cashews, and pistachios all contain 160 calories and 5 or 6 grams of protein per ounce. I suggest choosing the raw or dry roasted versions. I tend to stay away from peanut butters (which are actually a legume) because they grow underground and can carry a mold that can cause gastrointestinal problems for many. I also suggest reading labels and purchase a brand that contains as few ingredients as possible. I buy the brands that say: "nuts and maybe salt." I also would pass the ones up that contain hydrogenated oils or added sugar. Nut butters can be put onto bread, bananas, celery, apples and lots more for snacks!

- Sunflower and Sesame Seeds - a super healthy fat, these seeds contain significant protein in a small serving. Sunflower seeds contain the most protein @ 7.3 grams per quarter cup. Sesame seeds @ 5.4 grams per quarter cup. Always be thinking of how you can include seeds into your diet. I add them into salads and onto my avocado sandwich - smash the avocado and press some seeds onto it. I love them in soups for taste and garnish. Creating my own trail mix, I can add these wonderful seeds to it.

- Tempeh and Tofu – both of these are made from soybeans and have some of the highest vegetarian sources of protein. Both contain about 15 and 20 grams per half cup. The great part is that they are very nutritious, and will take on the taste and texture of whatever type of food you're looking to create. I purchase mine at my local health food store that has a variety. The firmer it is the more you can create dishes where you just substitute it for meat. A great stir-fry or appetizer is the most common way we use it in our household.

I created a raw high energy smoothie that we consume every morning after our lemon waters. One serving each, actually contains as much protein that we need in an entire day. Plant protein is easily absorbed and for those not liking greens, it's a great way to blend them up and get your greens in for the day!

Want one of the BEST secrets to experiencing healthy longevity? GREENS. Nothing comes close.

"If somebody's got beautiful skin,

it invites us to a deeper

understanding as to what is going on

inside their body."

~ David Wolfe

Chapter 21

What's The BIG Deal

About

Superfoods?

"Superfoods" is a term that has been used for the past 15+ years quite often. Exactly, what is a superfood and how important is incorporating several of them into your diet per day?

To sum it up, my personal definition of a "Superfood" is a food that your "cells love" and "respond well to." They are nutrient powerhouses that contain a variety of vitamins, minerals, polyphenols, anthocyanins, Omega-3 fatty acids and antioxidants depending on the superfood. They create an environment within our bodies that our immune systems and cells love to absorb and in turn become stronger and healthier each time one is consumed. It has been proven in hundreds of studies that these foods can reduce the risk of disease and prolong life. I believe that superfoods are a HUGE part of "The Edible Fountain of Youth Basket."

Beautiful skin along with looking young well into our 40's and beyond is what so many people around the world thrive for. They spend thousands of dollars per year on lotions and potions. As I said earlier in this book, a strong healthy plant based diet will do more for your skin from the inside out than anything else!

Three super foods I wanted to mention that I use very often and are exceptional for "our skin as we age" are:

Avocados, Berries and Green Tea:

1. Avocados

I believe, along with other experts, that an Avocado is a true superfood. They are rich in essential fatty acids which moisturize and feeds your skin. Because it contains B vitamins and vitamin E, it helps with elasticity and smoothness and the vitamin C builds up the layers of the skin which is what we all want. I usually consume 3-4 avocados per week (usually ½ per day) in a variety of ways. Just cut one up along with some fruit (apple, pear, etc.) for a great afternoon snack or use in the place of cheese on whole wheat crackers. I make avocado sandwiches and use it in a variety of wraps. Of course living in the southwest, homemade guacamole is a very common food to enjoy!

2. Berries

Berries of all kinds are FULL of antioxidants which kill free radicals and consequently prevents skin damage. If you are looking to have smooth, silky skin, berries can definitely help do this because they promote cell regeneration. The vitamin C is in abundance and helps feed the skin layers and internal structure. I consume blueberries every single day in my smoothie. This berry is a powerhouse when it comes to skin and anti-cancer protection. No matter what, get your berries in daily. You can put them on cereal, over salads, eat plain or into a smoothie. Endless possibilities if you like to bake.

3. Green Tea

Green tea contains so many antioxidants that drinking a cup or two (or more) per day is like putting money into your "health bank." It's been used as medicine for ages, so the research is in for it being classified as a superfood that enhances your health. I recommend green tea because of all the catechins it has in each and every cup which protects your skin from damage and free radicals. It's health benefits are numerous besides beautifying our largest organ. Green tea is proven to: improve brain function, helps kill cancer cells, boost your metabolism, reduces your risk of cardiac diseases and has shown anti-bacterial/anti-viral properties when exposed to bacteria and viruses. I would suggest trying green tea if you don't already love it. Each brand seems to have a little different flavor due to wherever it originated from, so give it a try. If no matter what you do not like green, other teas can be great tasting and effective too. Green tea rocks!

Here is a long list of "super healthy foods" I recommend, many of them are in the "superfood category", use as many of them per week as you can:

- Almonds, Almond Butter and Almond Milk – decrease cholesterol and improve heart health
- Asparagus – great for bones and a diuretic
- Avocados – super healthy fat, good for cardiac health
- Barley – lowers cholesterol
- Black Beans – protein for muscles and great for heart health
- Blueberries - improve memory, protects brain cells, heart health
- Broccoli Sprouts – major cancer preventing
- Brussels Sprouts – combats cancer and detoxifies
- Bok Choy – protects your bones
- Cauliflower – natural cancer fighter
- Cherries – antioxidants and blood vessels
- Collard greens – great for eye health
- Edamame – heart health, decrease inflammation and add fiber
- Farro – lowers cholesterol, keeps blood sugars stable
- Flaxseed – heart health, helps prevent some cancers
- Garlic – potent medicinal properties, heart and brain health
- Goji berries – skin, immune system and eye health

- Grapes (preferably red) heart-healthy resveratrol
- Grapefruit – immune system
- Herbs (sage, thyme, rosemary, oregano) heart health
- Lentils - major protein for healing
- Mushrooms (shiitake) – immune system and bone health
- Mustard Greens – major bone health and immune system
- Oats (whole) – great for cholesterol and heart health
- Oranges – immune system
- Rice (brown) – builds bones and converts food into energy
- Salmon – heart health and blood pressure
- Sardines – bone and heart health
- Spices – multiple health effects (see below)
- Spinach - helps blood clot and builds strong bones
- Strawberries – immune system may halt cancers
- Sunflower Seeds - heart healthy and fights infections
- Sweet Potatoes – protects vision, immune system, fiber
- Tea (green, black, white) – artery health and inflammation
- Tofu – protein and heart health
- Tomato (sauce) - skin look younger and heart health
- Oil – heart healthy (if no heart disease)

- Olives – heart health and skin
- Oranges – cholesterol and immune system
- Pumpkin (canned) – natural cancer fighter
- Walnuts - improve memory, coordination, heart health
- Wine (preferably red) – protect artery wall and cholesterol

Spices are also superfoods and a HUGE part of healthy aging. My kitchen cabinet is full of organic spices that not only make my meals taste great, they help to protect and improve my health.

In other countries and in many holistic practices in America, spices help to improve and prevent so many health issues. Between the essential oils and spices I have at my fingertips, I have the ability to enhance my health every single day.

Even though spices could be a chapter all its own, I want to talk about Turmeric. This one spice is in the news a lot lately, primarily because it has been studied intensely and the results are phenomenal of what it can do. The bright yellow pigment found in turmeric called "curcumin" (a polyphenol) is responsible for the majority of its medicinal properties and has over 600 potential health benefits.

The most important thing I wanted to pass on is that if you are using turmeric as a health promoter, be sure to use black pepper with it. The black pepper will increase its absorption rate by 2000%. Black pepper is actually added to curry powder.

In fact, if you want turmeric to remain in your body longer to benefit from its powerful effect, consume it with a healthy fat too. Turmeric is fat-soluble so it makes sense to do this. I add turmeric to my smoothie every morning because my nuts and ground flax are also in it. I do include a little black pepper to the mixture that is recommended to increase turmeric's absorption. When cooking with coconut oil, if the dish allows the flavor, add a little turmeric and black pepper for added health benefits. Do you always need a fat, to benefit from its powerful effects? No. It's just when a fat is added, the turmeric can be absorbed into the bloodstream through the lymphatic system thereby bypassing the liver. The positive effects stay in the body longer. But ALWAYS add the black pepper!

Brain health is an issue as we age. I am always looking how I can stay sharp and keep my brain healthy long into my 90's and beyond. Curcumin, found in the root of the turmeric plant, is one of the most powerful natural brain protecting substances on the planet. As we age, malformed proteins can form in the brain, when this happens the immune system sends out cells known as macrophages to engulf and destroy the proteins. If for some reason this function fails, non-healthy proteins accumulate in the brain and cognitive issues can develop.

Studies have shown that this yellow spice tends to encourage our immune systems to send macrophages to the brain, however, this amazing spice has the ability to pass into the brain, latch onto the beta-amyloid plaques and help the body break them down. Wow. What an impact it has on our brains. Turmeric is a daily spice used in my home for sure!

This is a long and not complete list (because it grows every day) of some of the disease processes that turmeric can positively impact.

Cardiovascular Disease, Cancer, Inflammatory Bowel Disease, Diabetes, Multiple Sclerosis, Metabolic Disease, Asthma, Allergies, Bronchitis, Neurodegenerative Diseases, Arthritis, Colitis, Nephrotoxicity, Cataracts, Wound Healing, Psoriasis and most, if not all, inflammatory diseases. Research turmeric and whatever health challenge you have and find out if you would benefit. I use it for prevention and healthy aging.

Bottom line, if you can add turmeric into your daily meals, it will definitely impact your health. Note, that if you are on any prescription medications, please check with your pharmacist to be sure that turmeric does not interfere with the drug's effectiveness.

"I do not think about being beautiful.

What I devote most of my time to

is being healthy."

~ Ann Bancroft

Chapter 22

The Health Benefits of

Organic Foods

Organic whole food products differ in their nutritional composition both in their raw and processed states. At a subjective level, this partially explains the differences in the sensory properties of food such as smell, texture and taste. Also, the numerous factors such as growing condition and season add to its advantages.

However, the opinion that organic food is healthier than conventional food is obviously a strong reason to consume it. Many people rally this part of healthy eating. It's the main reason why we have had a huge increase of growth in the organic food industry over the past 8-9 years because people have come to realize how important it is to make everything pertaining to what we put into our bodies as natural and pesticide free as possible.

Pesticides and fertilizer application have caused a lot of damages, particularly to the baby boomer generation and older, resulting in a multitude of disease processes being triggered by continuous exposures. On the other end of the spectrum are babies and children who easily absorb chemicals starting at birth. This is why many experts and myself believe that organic food is superior to other types.

First of all, there is scientific proof to show that many organic foods are better than conventional or orthodox food. The Environmental Working Group has a website with this particular article along with others to enhance your knowledge.

(http://www.ewg.org/foodnews/summary.php)

It goes much more into detail about what we are exposed to and how we can make good choices.

Many people don't understand what the BIG DEAL is about eating as much organic as we can. Realize that our world has changed drastically in the past 15-20 years with processed foods and chemical exposures more than any time in history. Wanting to do whatever you can to avoid serious disease while aging well means you need to pay attention to the chemicals that surround you.

This information is from their website, for additional info please visit the link posted above and below:

Highlights of Dirty Dozen™ 2015

EWG singles out produce with the highest pesticide loads for its Dirty Dozen™ list. This year, it is comprised of apples, peaches, nectarines, strawberries, grapes, celery, spinach, sweet bell peppers, cucumbers, cherry tomatoes, imported snap peas and potatoes.

Each of these foods tested positive a number of different pesticide residues and showed higher concentrations of pesticides than other produce items.

Key findings:

99 percent of apple samples, 98 percent of peaches, and 97 percent of nectarines tested positive for at least one pesticide residue.

The average potato had more pesticides by weight than any other produce.

A single grape sample and a sweet bell pepper sample contained 15 pesticides.

Single samples of cherry tomatoes, nectarines, peaches, imported snap peas and strawberries showed 13 different pesticides apiece.

EWG's Clean Fifteen™ *list of produce least likely to hold pesticide residues consists of avocados, sweet corn, pineapples, cabbage, frozen sweet peas, onions, asparagus, mangoes, papayas, kiwis, eggplant, grapefruit, cantaloupe, cauliflower and sweet potatoes. Relatively few pesticides were detected on these foods, and tests found low total concentrations of pesticides on them.*

Key findings:

Avocados were the cleanest: only 1 percent of avocado samples showed any detectable pesticides.

Some 89 percent of pineapples, 82 percent of kiwi, 80 percent of papayas, 88 percent of mango and 61 percent of cantaloupe had no residues.

No single fruit sample from the Clean Fifteen™ *tested positive for more than 4 types of pesticides.*

Multiple pesticide residues are extremely rare on Clean Fifteen™ *vegetables. Only 5.5 percent of Clean Fifteen samples had two or more pesticides.*

If you are a parent or grandparent I suggest you read their article about the exposures in baby foods. And if you are on a budget and cannot afford some organic food items, stick to the Clean 15 as much as you can to lower your risk along with your family's risk. A knowledgeable consumer is a healthier consumer!!!

Antioxidant capacity: A number of studies carried out have shown that antioxidants tend to have more of a boost when they come from organic foods and eaten within a few days right off the vine. This may be due to the fact that foreign chemicals from processed foods negatively interacts with the different minerals. Vitamins that are supposed to positively impact fruits and vegetables to prevent challenges like cancer, heart diseases, premature aging, cognitive malfunction and vision problems are immediately available. Recent research proves that choosing organic foods will lead to increased intake of nutritionally desirable antioxidants and a much less exposure, if at all, to heavy metals.

Heart health: Anything good for our aging brain is good for our heart.   Conjugated linoleic acid happens to be a heart- healthy fatty acid that can enhance cardiovascular protection, and also prevents any related heart disease. There are high levels of anti-oxidants in organic fruits and vegetables, decreasing inflammation which can decrease cardiac events.

Overall health: Since organic food is not prepared using chemical enrichers, it means it does not contain any of these strong chemicals and will not affect the human body in negative ways, unlike the application of pesticides to non-organic foods. These pesticides contain powerful chemicals like organophosphorus that may cause potential developmental problems like autism and ADHD in children and adults.

Since harmful chemicals are not applied to organic foods while growing, the environment will be free from any form of pollution. This is important as we want to leave our children's children with a healthy field of dirt not harmed by years of chemical exposure.

Here is a video link to a beautiful family, just like yours, whose blood levels were taken **before** and **after** a 2-week session of eating organics. I am sure that you will want to see this. It's only 1min, 32 secs long.

http://www.foodmatters.tv/content/the-organic-effect-a-short-documentary

"If we focus on our health, including

our inner health,

our self-esteem, how we look at ourselves

and our confidence level,

we'll tend to be healthier people.

We'll tend to make better choices

for our lives, for our bodies and

we'll always be trying to learn more and

get better as time goes on."

~ Queen Latifah

Chapter 23

Lemon Water

Detox

And

Liver Cleansing

Want a kick start to your morning? Want to get your digestion going first thing? One of my favorite habits to enjoy as I rise in the morning (besides journaling in my gratitude journal and meditating) is drinking lemon water in a glass of room temperature filtered water. It has become a part of my daily routine and it has made a huge difference for me. Lemon water has an incredible amount of health benefits.

Lemon's Health Benefits:

- Aging skin can benefit because lemons are an excellent source of antioxidant which prevents free radical damage causing pre-mature aging of your skin.
- It increases and maintains your skins elasticity. Vitamin C fruits helps to prevent wrinkles and create a smoother looking skin.
- Great for brain and nerve health. If you lead a busy lifestyle or a stressed life,

adding a glass of lemon water daily will allow you to focus more.

- It's a digestive aid and liver cleanser. Helps ease indigestion, bloating and heartburn.
- Hydrates your colon and helps you move your bowels. Vital for a healthy life – "what goes in must come out." Longer your stool remains in your body, the more it can cause havoc to our system.
- As we age, our joints can build up uric acid. Lemons have the ability to remove it and decrease inflammation.
- It has a strong antibacterial, antiviral, and immune-boosting powers which as we age is huge.
- Lemons are very alkalizing. An acidic body attracts illness and disease. An alkalized body can slow the aging process and maintain health much longer.
- Lemons improve the ability to absorb iron from the foods we eat.
- Boosts your energy and can improve your mood.
- Lemons contain so many good nutrients such as calcium, magnesium, vitamin C, citric acid, bioflavonoids, pectin. All of these work towards promoting immunity and fighting infection. You are boosting your immune system every day you drink lemon water.

- Stimulates your liver to produce more enzymes which then flushes out toxins in your tissues, organs and cells.

I purchase only organic fresh lemons if possible. If you cannot, be sure to wash the lemons well before cutting open. Never use processed lemon juice for your morning cleanse. I squeeze ½ of a large lemon (if small, then a whole one) into a glass of warm or room temperature water and literally drink it down first thing before I enjoy my breakfast raw smoothie.

Recently, I have been buying organic lemons when they are on sale, cleaning them well, removing the skin and any seeds and putting them directly into my NutriBullet. Then I pour the blended lemons into a non-BPA ice tray and freeze for 24 hours. After they are frozen, I pop them out into a bag and keep them in the freezer. Then if I do not have any fresh lemons at home, I take out 1-2 frozen cubes placing them into a tall glass, add room temp or warm water as they melt pretty quickly and enjoy. My liver thanks me every morning! Quick and easy. This is such an easy "healthy aging" tip to do!

"Every time you eat or drink, you are either feeding disease or fighting it."

~ Heather Morgan

Chapter 24

Cooking with Essential Oils

Essential oils are absolutely fascinating to cook with and have been used in the cooking process for thousands of years. Cooking with essential oils consist of drops filled with vibrant oils which can flavor a dish to your liking. Not only can they enhance your cuisine, they can enhance your health as well. If you are willing to learn how to include essential oils into your meals, you can improve your body from the inside out while making it a part of your healthy aging plan.

Plants were our original medicine and in some countries, they still are commonly used. Today, pharmaceutical synthetic medications are what most people are familiar with. Plants work on a holistic level and can be very effective. The essential oils I use cost pennies per day versus what medications cost.

I believe that with the right oils, it can become a game changer for the healthy dishes you prepare. I will be teaching more about "Cooking with Essential Oils" as part of my series of classes.

There are four main oil groups to cook with:

Spices, Herbs, Flowers and Citrus Fruits!

These oils with enhance the flavor of any dish you are preparing. Everything from soups to sauces, desserts to cakes, the ideas are endless.

FYI: Not all essential oils can be ingested. Synthetic oils should NOT be taken internally and should not be ingested. Read the labels carefully because plant medicine is potent and not all of the essential oils are meant to be taken internally. Certified pure therapeutic grade oils is the best in the industry. Be very picky where you buy them.

Learn more about *Essential Oils* on my website:

www.TheEdibleFountainOfYouth.com

I will share with you the type of oils and the brand that I use, which is the best of the best.   I believe once you learn how to incorporate these healthy oils into your favorite dishes you will be including them in your "edible fountain of youth basket" to cook with!

"Look up, laugh loud, talk big, keep the

color in your cheeks and the

fire in your eye, adorn your person,

maintain your health, your beauty

and your animal spirits."

~ William Hazlitt

Chapter 25

Red Wine,

Dark Chocolate

and

Aging Well

Many adults are just as excited about wine as they are about dark chocolate! First, if you are not a drinker, don't start just because wine is safe and healthy in small amounts. But for those who appreciate a glass a day, this will be good, no "GREAT" news. Wine really rocks when it comes to helping us age gracefully.

According to WebMD, (a very reputable source) they interviewed Richard A. Baxter, MD, a plastic surgeon in Seattle and then shared his "wine wisdom" with their followers. They asked Dr. Baker, what is it about wine that can help us age and look better?

This is what he said...

"There is quite a lot of data on the wine and beauty connection. I was surprised at how extensive the data is on wine as an antiaging intervention."

"The mechanism is the antioxidants in red wine. Antioxidants sop up damaging free radicals that play a role in aging and age-related diseases. There is a much higher concentration of antioxidants called polyphenols, including resveratrol, in wine compared to grape juice. In wine, the skin and seeds are part of the fermenting process, but both are removed when making grape juice."

"I think stress has something to do with it, too. It is difficult to sort out how much of the benefits are from the chemical properties of wine vs. the types of behaviors that wine drinkers tend to have such as less stress in their lives. Wine is part of the Mediterranean diet, which is also rich in fresh fruits and vegetables, whole grains, nuts and seeds, legumes, seafood, yogurt, and olive oil. This diet is more of a lifestyle that includes drinking wine with dinner. Studies show that the Mediterranean diet is associated with longer, healthier lives."

"Drinking a glass of red wine a day is the single most important thing that you can do other than nonsmoking, from an antiaging point of view, but you can have too much of a good thing. Drinking more than recommended can have the opposite effect on your appearance and health."

By Dr. Richard A. Baxter

Author of 'Age Gets Better with Wine'

Here is a list of benefits that I personally have studied and found to be true:

Wine...

- Lowers your risk for blood clots
- Helps increase your HDL (good cholesterol)
- Great for your brain especially as we age
- Reduces pre-cancerous skin lesions
- Benefits our cardiac system promoting better arterial function
- Lowers the risk of prostate cancer for men.
- It's a common desire to look younger and wine can really impact our aging skin

Red wine studies have been shown to slow down the aging process. How does it do that? Red wine contains a number of compounds called flavonoids. One compound called resveratrol measures high in red wine. That's what gives it the red color and literally can help stop the early signs of aging. Red wine is also rich in anti-oxidants which destroy harmful free radicals in our bodies. There are also enzymes in wine that help with cell regeneration.

How much wine is beneficial to drink?

Experts recommend 4-5 oz. for women and 8-9 oz. for men. Drink more than that on a regular basis and it definitely can turn from a healthy enjoyment to setting yourself up for health challenges.

Because I enjoy wine and it has proven heart health benefits, I sip on a 4-ounce glass of Pinot Noir a couple nights a week. Pinot Noir rocks when it comes to having an anti-aging phytonutrient called resveratrol in it. Several studies have found that Pinot Noir is richer in resveratrol than most wines. So since I want to maximize my heart healthy benefits with everything I eat and drink, Pinot Noir fills my wine rack.

Enjoy your glass of resveratrol, CHEERS!

Want to slow down the aging process AND enjoy it along the way? **Chocolate is one of those attractive foods that people LOVE** to hear is good for us. The skin protecting properties of dark chocolate makes it a super healthy aging food. Dark chocolate does contain flavonoids which helps keep our skin soft along with protecting it from the sun's harmful rays. Dark chocolate can help reduce high blood pressure and lower your "bad" cholesterol (also known as LDL).

WorldHealth.net is a very reputable website that represents 26,000 physicians and scientists from 120 countries worldwide. They wrote an article about chocolate and several studies that were done on this decadent antioxidant. After reading them, I wanted to include two of the studies in this chapter to make you understand the powerful properties in dark chocolate.

"A team from University of Milan (Italy) assessed the effect of a dark chocolate composed of 860 mg polyphenols and containing 58 mg epicatechin, a specific type of antioxidant polyphenol. The team assigned 20 healthy men and women, average age 24.2 years, to consume a balanced diet for 4 weeks, midway through which one-half of the subjects were asked to additionally consume dark chocolate. The researchers observed that catechin levels increased just two hours after the consumption of the dark chocolate, a rise that coincidentally correlated to decreases in DNA damage on the order of 20% that were observed in blood cells."

The second study - "Researchers from the Laboratory of Genetic and Environmental Epidemiology at Catholic University (Italy) studied a group of 5,000 subjects in generally good health over a one-year period. Specifically, the evaluated the anti-inflammatory properties of dark chocolate, as measured by serum levels of C-reactive protein (CRP), a blood marker of inflammation. The team found that those subjects who consumed 1 serving (20 g) of dark chocolate every 3 days had serum CRP concentrations that were significantly lower than those who did not eat any chocolate. According to the researchers, these reductions in CRP translate to a 33% risk reduction of cardiovascular disease in women and 26% reduction in men."

WOW. What is the secret in the chocolate bar? It is not the sugar, in fact when consuming it, read the label if you are doing it for your health and be sure there is more than 70% cacao which will give you the best results. Twenty grams twice a week is what they recommend, to improve your cardiovascular risk profile.

If you can find raw cacao, it is extremely high in an ORAC rating, meaning it is substantially better that red wine or blueberries. Cacao is also high in essential fatty acids and become a great anti-inflammatory food.

Please read the back of the bar for specific serving sizes. Remember, when you consume chocolate under 70% cacao and increase the amount of sugars, you can encourage inflammation and counteract what the chocolate can do for you.

I suggest purchasing the large bars of organic chocolate and placing them in glass covered jars to keep fresh. I enjoy a small piece of dark chocolate with a cup of hot green tea or 4 oz. of pinot noir wine and get a double whammy of antioxidants!!!

Relax and enjoy...

"Walking is magic.

Can't recommend it highly enough.

I read that Plato and Aristotle

did much of their brilliant thinking

together while ambulating.

The movement, the meditation, the health

of the blood pumping, and the

rhythm of footsteps...

this is a primal way to connect with

one's deeper self."

~ Paula Cole

Chapter 26

Moving for Longevity

Exercise

+

Eating Well

=

A Long Healthy Life!

Exercise. The dreaded word for many. An addiction for some. My suggestion: become addicted to feeling good and looking well and exercise can help you get there faster. Exercising for prevention is the name of the game, however, if you have health challenges and want some serious improvement, then exercise has to be incorporated into your daily routine because it can and will change things around for you.

What is the best exercise? Is joining a gym better than working out at home? Should I join a class? How often should I exercise? What if I don't like to exercise? It's boring, it hurts, I am tired when I wake up, I am rushed after work, I don't have time, and I don't have money.

My answer is...do whatever kind of exercise that will get you to move. For some, it's the treadmill and weights, for others it's an aerobic dance class or power walking. You can create or join a group of walkers who inspire each other. Do WHATEVER you can to MOVE and move DAILY!

I want you to take what I am saying to heart, so let's look at life as if it changed drastically for you today. This particular scenario I have seen dozens of times in my 30+ year career. I hope this never happens to you but hopefully you will see why I am adamant about eating well AND exercising daily.

This is a real story of one of my patient I treated in 2012. He was only 52. It could be you. Picture yourself in this serious situation a couple years from now because you continued consuming poor food choices with little to no exercise and out of control stress management.

You have been admitted to the hospital after having a serious heart attack where you were saved by paramedics who shocked your heart after several minutes of you being without a heartbeat. Because of the damage, you now only have 20% heart function left and the doctors tell your family that you are extremely lucky to be alive. You are hooked up to all kind of wires, an oxygen mask over your nose and mouth and you are now on 6 different medications you weren't on yesterday.

The doctor tells you that YOUR life will be limited now, you will easily become short of breath, will not be able to return to work *and life will be very different as you knew it.* Over the next few days, as reality sets in, you discuss with your family the cost of being ill and realize that your medications along with the high deductible insurance you have may exceed $5000 each and every year.

Wow. You lie there in disbelief. Wishing you could go back a year or two – you may have considered eating much better, including more antioxidants on a daily basis; perhaps less sugars and animal products and increased the amount of plant based foods into your diet. You may have worked on your stress level more, learning different techniques to calm the inflammation within your organs that stress influences. You may have joined a gym, going often and putting up with temporary muscle pain, making the time and energy into your daily schedule. Perhaps you would pay the $40-month gym fee, realizing that a years' membership fee is far less than even a day in the hospital. Sad part is, you cannot go back. Again, what we do today we pay for tomorrow – good or bad.

"Sleep is that golden chain that ties

health and our bodies together."

~ Thomas Dekker

"Early to bed and early to rise

makes a man

healthy, wealthy and wise."

~ Benjamin Franklin

Chapter 27

Poor Habits That "Attract Disease"

and

"Speed the Aging Process"

- *Sedentary lifestyle and lack of exercise:*

  Did you know that exercise increases blood flow throughout the entire body, making you feel and look healthier? Most people do not have to partake in strenuous exercise for optimal health. Any moderate aerobic physical activity for at least thirty minutes every day will have a positive impact on your health. Remember, anything that benefits your heart and brain will benefit you as you age. Start today, build yourself up. Don't fool yourself that you can skip this part!

If you have a job that requires you to sit for more than 2 hours straight at a time, get up and stretch or walk around when you can. Movement throughout the day is so vital to your weight along with your cardiac and musculoskeletal system. Set your alarm or get some type of Fitbit like device.

I power walk in the morning for 45 minutes and if home for the day, I set my alarm for every 60-90 minutes, take a break and walk on my treadmill another 9-12 minutes each time. By the end of the day, I have reached my 10k steps and decreased the amount of sedentary time that could age my body or influence disease. If I have a crazy busy work day outside of my home, then I try to get in a couple longer walking sessions. Do I enjoy exercising? ...actually no I don't. But I definitely want the results of a fit and healthy body and mind. Gotta do what you gotta do!!!

- *Smoking:*

It's certainly no news that smoking is bad for your health. It's even written on the cigarette packs, but did you know it affects your looks too? Studies have shown that in addition to shortening your life (by increasing your risk for lung and heart disease), smoking can set off and trigger enzymes that can break down the layers of your skin.

The skin is your largest organ and needs oxygen to maintain its structure. Most people can spot a smoker by looking at their skin and then listening to them whenever they cough. Smoker's tend to look much older than their chronological age no matter how many lotions they use. There are a many options available for quitting this habit. If your goal is long term health and want to really enjoy longevity – get help today.

- *Crash dieting*:

Crash dieting is never a good idea, it's more of a long term threat than a long term or short term solution. Crash dieting makes you feel older by reducing your energy level, slowing your metabolism, fluctuating your concentration and can cause depression. Crash dieting can cause electrolyte disturbances in some people which will affect their cardiac status.

Aging skin does not have time to adjust to fast weight loss. Lose, then gain, lose, then gain = stretched skin and lost elasticity. So clearly, you are posing a great danger to your overall health by crash dieting without a positive outcome. I suggest developing a healthy eating "lifestyle" and with all the changes, the weight will come off. You will be much happier and it's a long term solution.

Find help if you need it. There are excellent nutritionists and dieticians along with doctors and nurses who specialize in weight loss. Find one who not only has the credentials but looks like they practice what they preach. Please be aware of the people who call themselves "nutrition experts" and sell diet products. Remember, if it sounds too good to be true, it probably is. Look for credentials. I do not recommend any diet pills, patches, drinks or "miracle supplements". Most do not work and even if they did on a short term basis, they are not a long term fix - either from a health standpoint or financially hitting your pocketbook hard and then you quit. Learning to eat well from your local grocers is a much better solution. Lifestyle is the answer to everything as we age.

- *Lack of Adequate Sleep*:

When we sleep our cells regenerate, our organs refresh themselves and our brains rest and renew. Most people think they don't need much sleep. However, the truth is, studies have shown that we all need at least seven to eight hours every night, especially for long term health. If you don't get enough sleep, it reduces your effectiveness during the day with driving, your job, relationships and your health. Studies have shown that without a good sleeping pattern you can age your brain quicker, irritating certain areas in the brain that can bring on dementia. Whoa, not good.

If you possibly have sleep apnea and if left untreated can cause a person to invite several health issues into their lives (strokes, heart attacks, weight gain, high cortisol levels, internal inflammation, etc.).

If you sleep with a "snorer" and they keep you awake, your health is danger too. YOU need quality sleep, period. They need to be evaluated by their medical practitioner and if they are concerned, have a sleep study. Then if you do not have sleep apnea, visit your dentist or an ENT physician for a mouth piece you can wear at night. Seriously, there is mounting research about the dangers of poor sleeping habits. Plus, the lack of quality sleep will age you faster.

- *Sunscreens*:

  Spending time outside without sunscreens is asking for aging skin. I'm sure this is not your first time reading about this, yet many of you ignore the suggestions because you think it isn't necessary, or the minutes you spend outside doesn't hurt or promote aging. Wrong.

  Unprotected sun exposure can cause significant damage in the future like skin cancer and it certainly can accelerate the rate of aging. Remember, skin cancer takes years to show itself. Once it does it can spread rapidly throughout your other organs.

  Put a hat on. Use sunscreen or clothing to decrease exposure. Many companies put sunscreen in their makeup products which is great, however, if you are at the beach or just outdoors for any length of time, you still need to reapply sunscreen every hour or so. The SPF in most makeup is 15. More than 30 is best for the face. Staying out of the sun while it is at its peak is recommended. Wear sunglasses to protect your eyes and avoid sunburns for yourself and for your children. What you do to your skin today, you will pay for tomorrow, good or bad.

- *Overzealous cleansing and not being in the habit of skin brushing:*

Some cleansers that are applied to our delicate skin are made with harsh ingredients, thus stripping the skin of its natural oil that keeps it supple. Get to know your skin type, and apply cleansers/creams that suit it. Alcohol in products can dry your skin out even if it is in a lotion. Don't exfoliate with cleansers made for teens if you are not a teen. There are so many great products out there that will make you feel and smell clean but not strip your skin of the oils it needs for good health. Treat your skin well.

Dry skin brushing is a health habit you can start tomorrow and benefit from right away. Skin brushing is a powerful detoxification aid. It's a fantastic way to promote circulation. When you brush your dry skin, (perhaps prior to your shower), your blood flow increases and the normal process of releasing toxins is improved. Incorporating this habit can also improve digestion, kidney function and decrease stress.

The biggest reason I skin brush, besides getting rid of dry skin and improving my circulation, is really it helps my lymphatic system. This incredible cleansing system is responsible for eliminating cellular waste products in your body. When it is not working properly, waste and toxins can build up and create issues and illness. Stimulating your skin with a dry brush helps to release toxins, therefore, decreases inflammation.

If you have never dry skin brushed yourself, here is some easy instructions to follow.

Purchase a natural bristle brush, NOT a synthetic one. Get one with a long handle so you can reach all areas on your body.

- Remove all your clothes and step into shower or bathtub to catch the skin flakes. I know this sounds gross but dead skin needs to come off and if you do not skin brush, then your clothes will eventually catch it all without the benefit.
- Starting at the bottom with your dry brush, *take long strokes up towards the heart,* do not go away from the heart, *move towards it.*
- Brush each and every area. Be gentle around tender skin. Use light pressure. You should NOT see red marks, just perhaps light pink skin from your circulation being stimulated.

- Take about 5-10 minutes to complete the process, then jump into the shower.
- You may want to apply a lotion or oil upon getting out of the warm shower!

Last but not least, drink lots of water and stay out of really warm/hot showers that may dry you out. Your beautiful skin will thank you!

- *Stress and worrying too much:*

    Constant or frequent worry and stress can age us quickly. The internal buildup of cortisol and inflammation within our organs can be huge. This undoubtedly is asking for health issues to arise. Try as much as possible not to let it interfere with your life and your health.

    I'm sure you have seen or heard of how stress affects us all. Literally thousands of studies have been done on stress and its effects on your body. Stress can cause high blood pressure, stroke and multiple other diseases. They estimate that over 90% of all doctor office visits are a result of stress on the body which triggers illness. I'm sure you don't want to experience how stress can wreak havoc on both your mental and physical health.

    Are you the type of person that worries too much? Do you stress yourself over irrelevant things? If yes, perhaps you are taking life's ups and downs too seriously. Undoubtedly, you are speeding up the aging process. Learning to manage it is possible. So much can be done, but you have to reach out. Get help, it's all around you. A great life coach or therapist can help you put things into perspective. Meditate. Journal. Make a decision today that you will not let stress harm your health, speed up your aging process and/or attract disease.

- *Poor eating habits:*

  This book is all about living and aging well. If you have read this book so far then you know that improving your eating habits can be absolutely the best longevity plan... today, tomorrow and in the future.

  When you, by choice, (yes it is a choice) don't consume enough fruits and vegetables, then you are encouraging the multitude of activities that antioxidants do including prevent oxidative stress caused by free radicals. It's well known that free radicals can damage every single cell within your body. Since you are reading this book, you are obviously looking for help to improve your health. EAT YOUR VEGGIES.

You do not want to be one of the - "could of, would of, should of people" I talked about in earlier chapters. Take it seriously and make a commitment to your future.

- *Strong relationships*:

  Studies have shown that having great relationships is vital to surviving well as we age. Having someone to count on, to laugh and cry with, to help you through the thick and thin of life is so very important.

  You may look at your current circle of "influencers" -> family and friends who influence how you eat, drink, handle finances, take care of yourself, exercise, handle stress, etc. and decide that this year you are going to expand your circle to people who are living well, eating healthy, enjoying life and decreasing their stress. We truly are a sum of the people in our circle.

  Reach out, join a club, find friends on Facebook who you can share your life happenings with. Do whatever you need to. Find a few positive "influencers" and your life will change for the better.

  And SMILE each and every day – it helps extend your blessed life.

- *Avoiding IMPORTANT health exams:*

This would be like never performing preventative care on your car. Never having the oils, belts, motor and engine checked. Eventually the chances of something happening is huge.

Respect your body, you only have one. A scheduled health checkup should be done yearly or for many biannually - or you may be asking for trouble. Even if you feel good and look good. Find a primary care provider who understands preventative medicine, nutrition and healthy living. Then you should schedule to see them. You can talk about health issues, concerns or ask questions. You will have your vitals checked, heart and lungs listened to by a trained ear, routine labs to see what is going on internally and then review them. It's the labs that change slowly over time that alerts your practitioner that something may be brewing inside and to take action or monitor it closely.

Having your vision checked is so important every 2 years and more often for those with possible eye disease, diabetes or if you are instructed to. Having an issue, then scheduling an exam is not smart when it comes to your eyes. Prevention or finding issues early is vital.

For those over 50 or for those in a high risk category, scheduling a colonoscopy is imperative. For the ladies, definitely a good GYN visit and mammogram until that doctor tells you you've reached the age you do not need them anymore.

"If you don't think your anxiety,

depression, sadness and stress

impact your physical health,

think again. All of these emotions trigger

chemical reactions in your body,

which can lead to inflammation and a

weakened immune system.

Learn how to cope, sweet friend.

There will always be darker days."

~ Kris Carr

Chapter 28

Hormonal Imbalance
As We Age

Hormone imbalance has been heavily advertised as the reason why we age. It's true that our hormones affect every single thing we do; our body is run by hormones. However, it is just one of the many reasons we may age faster or with many challenges.

Signs/symptoms of

hormonal changes for <u>WOMEN</u>:

Bone loss - osteopenia and/or osteoporosis

Wrinkles and skin elasticity issues

Skin issues, dryness, wrinkles

Brain Fog

Weight Gain

Mood swings

Perimenopause

Premenstrual Syndrome

Menopause

Depression

Loss of energy

Hot Flashes

Irritability

Bloating

Night Sweats

Low Libido

Insomnia

Signs/symptoms of

hormonal changes for MEN:

Erectile Dysfunction

Heart disease

Loss of strength

Loss of energy

Insomnia

Low sex drive

Weight gain

Andropause

Depression

There is so much great information and I suggest you speak with a well-qualified physician who specializes in "aging hormonal changes." Getting the correct blood work to create a baseline for treatment is essential. There is A LOT of products out there on the internet that are NOT good for most of us. Because it's a huge industry, lots of scammers can call themselves medical professional and aren't.

When it comes to your hormones, if you decide to buy a product, I HIGHLY suggest you check out their credentials and possible run it past your doctor. I believe that you should be seen by a specialist if you have symptoms. Ads online do not replace a face to face visit. Problems can arise. Screwing with your hormones is not a great idea without the knowledge. The products may or may not work for you, you may waste your $$ or worse yet, they may harm you. Without baseline tests you are taking a shot in the dark.

For women, if you want to read some great information about hormones, I suggest Dr. Christiane Northrup's books. She is a very credible physician with much experience and her book can help guide you to your next step. You can find her books on Amazon.

"Laughter is the best medicine"

~ a proverb from the wisdom of Solomon.

Chapter 29

Laughter, Relationships
and Healthy Aging

Even though this book focuses on the "edible" part of healthy aging, I cannot leave out laughter and the bonds we have in life.

Do whatever you can to laugh out loud a few times per day! When you mix laughter, super healthy foods, friendship and family around a grand table - you have hit the health jackpot! How important is laughter in our baskets of youth? Tremendously important.

Laughter is necessary for having a high degree of health into your 70's, 80's and beyond. It can relax your whole body and relieve physical tension and stress. Studies have shown that

Centenarians (those who lives to or beyond the age of 100 years) have had years and years of laughter and a support system in their lives.

Some of the health benefits of laughter are: It can improve your immune system, your mood and stimulates many organs by releasing endorphins (feel good hormones). It can soothe tension and can help relieve pain and healing.

For those of you that are limited to people who can put a smile on your face, I suggest going to YouTube and watching little kids do funny things, or better yet, adults doing silly or funny things. Also, pets can easily put a smile on your face. I have patients who record the "Ellen" show and get their daily laughter in at the end of a long day. Bottom line, laughter is a huge part of keeping your brain and heart young. Laughter is known as one of the very BEST medicines!

Relationships and deep social connections have proven to keep not only our hearts sound but our brains healthier. These two topics have been researched thousands of times and the end result is always the same. *Your life is the sum of relationships you have.* I have pointed it out before but it's that important. *Your circle of friends is an important part of your life!*

Here is a short video clip that will point out the importance of "relationships" as we grow into our beautiful lives.

http://www.ted.com/talks/robert_waldinger_what_makes_a_good_life_lessons_from_the_longest_study_on_happiness

"Your body will be around for a lot longer

than that expensive handbag.

Invest in yourself."

~ Unknown Author

Chapter 30

Are You Ready to Take
YOUR Health
to the Next Level
&
Get Started?

You have one body, one soul and one mind. You are never too old to set another goal or to dream a new dream. You are never too old to improve or strengthen your health. Correcting it sooner than later is the smartest action to take. I say this for those who are afraid that it's too late to have a healthy lifestyle or rid themselves of their health challenges and multiple medications.

Look in the mirror and ask yourself, am I ready? If not today, then when? *Procrastination with our health fills up hospitals, clinics and graveyards.*

This is not a diet book. It's a healthy aging lifestyle book where you have the information and now you need to move forward. There comes a time in everyone's life when they wake up and realize that their daily health decisions have affected their tomorrows. We are never guaranteed our health.

How different or better would your life be if you felt better? Had more energy? Lost weight? Decreased the inflammation in your body? What could you do if your health did not stop you from accomplishing it?

Get started TODAY. Figure out what stopped you in the past and then don't go back there! Start by really getting to know your body. Journaling during this process can be important especially if you are working with someone who can help you through the issues that may arise. A health/life coach, nutritionist or medical practitioner is suggested. I definitely had my patients keeping journals. First, tracking your food consumption can help to really see what you are putting into your engine. But what is equally as important is your feelings and any issues you have as you moved forward.

Changing dietary habits can be a breeze for some people but the majority of us will have some challenges. Over the years, poor habits have become imbedded into our subconscious minds creating health and dietary choices, good and bad. Good news – you can change that for the better starting NOW. Know that everything you do today, will affect your tomorrows.

Here are 9 things I suggest you do every day as you get started on your venture towards exceptional health!

- Start with a positive attitude that *healthy aging is important to you*, this will create and set the tone for your desired benefits. Start a vision board. If you can see it, you can achieve it. Put positive messages to yourself all around your home or at least on your bathroom mirror. Hang around those who will support you on your quest, very important.

- Move every day. Exercise without any excuses. I prefer power walking with some strength training for extra bone health and to not lose precious muscle. (Refer back to the chapter on exercising for longevity).

- Schedule at least 7-8 hours of sleep at night. If that's not possible then a 15-minute power nap in the afternoon is needed. Our body's need to refill, our cells need to regenerate and only sleep can give us that. Sleep is a healthy aging secret!

- Drink at least 64 ounces of filtered water every day unless advised by your primary care provider to do more or less. Great for skin, your kidneys, weight loss, metabolism and much more. Coffee is such a loved beverage but start looking at what you are adding to each cup. The calories add up quickly and the sugar content can increase your blood sugar along with cellular inflammation. Multiple studies have shown that coffee beans are definitely healthy, but if it causes you to sleep poorly, then go for decaf or teas without caffeine after 12 noon. If you have learned anything, it's *your cells rule your internal world.*" Happy cells, happy life!

- Record and look at your stools. Sounds odd, however, your gut and bowel health is vital especially as you age. The majority of people should have a BM at least once per day. When you consume the typical SAD diet, there may not be enough fiber to push things through on a regular basis. What goes in must come out, right? Ridding yourself of the toxins is vital. If your diet was filled with processed foods, then getting the residue out as soon as possible is a step forward. Probiotics such as acidophilus will help along with ground flaxseeds (I put mine in my smoothie every day). Trust me, if you start adding in more fiber, your stools will increase and you will see a healthy outcome in your toilet...yeah.

- Eat a clean, plant based diet avoiding processed foods and meats. Consume as many vegetables as possible with a couple servings of fruit per day. If you remain eating animal protein, become informed of what is the safest (not processed meats like hotdogs) to consume and what's the best and safest way to cook it. Just be sure it's a small serving and organic if possible. Initially, cruciferous veggies would be my list to help with your detox. Some examples are: cabbage, brussel sprouts, kale and broccoli. Adding some garlic and onions will help too. Then add as many superfoods into your weekly menu.

- Meditate. Not sure where to start? YouTube.com has some great meditation videos. Oprah has put together (along with Deepak Chopra) meditations that are phenomenal. You can find the link on her website: www.Oprah.com We all need to shut our minds down for peace, refresh our brains and gain overall health. There are proven studies showing the long term effect of meditation. Daily rituals are a huge part of my anti-aging lifestyle.

- Find someone to share your healthy aging program with. It may increase your chances of success if you can share the process. Again, it is very important hang around those who will support you on your journey. Learn all you can from *reputable* authorities. Avoid dietary and nutritional "wanna be" scammers.

- Whether you eat animal protein or not, I suggest buying a vegetarian or vegan cookbook and/or perhaps a plant based diet magazine. Why? We all know how to cook meats, the reason most Americans do not eat a variety of vegetables, beans, legumes and rice is that they have NO idea what to do with them. Make the meat your side dish and find some great recipes for your plant based main dish.

- Clean out your cupboards. If you can afford to give away the items that advance aging or shorten your life, then do it. Again, think about the car with bad gas – how many of you would take a chance putting in bad gas because it was on sale? Toss it. Make the decision today to take part in your ability to create a super healthy body that ages slowly and with great energy and unbelievable health.

Conclusion

Health is just a decision...

We cannot change our chronological age. I cannot stop myself nor any of my patients or loved ones from aging. What I can do is teach, motivate and inspire those interested to live well.

By you participating in the future of your health, you will not only extend your lifespan but may live with much more passion, love and vibrant health than you could of ever imagine!

Now that you are done with this book, ask yourself - what information did I really grasp and throw into my 'Edible Fountain of Youth Basket?'

Recipes can be found in Susan's new cookbook

"Eat the Way YOU Want to Look" ™

to be released in early 2016. It is filled with her own delicious health busting recipes along with those that she highly recommends and have used for many years.

Follow Susan on Facebook and on her website

www.TheEdibleFountainOfYouth.com

to learn about upcoming seminars, webinars, cooking classes and tips to live an amazingly healthy lifestyle!